Sonography Study Notebook

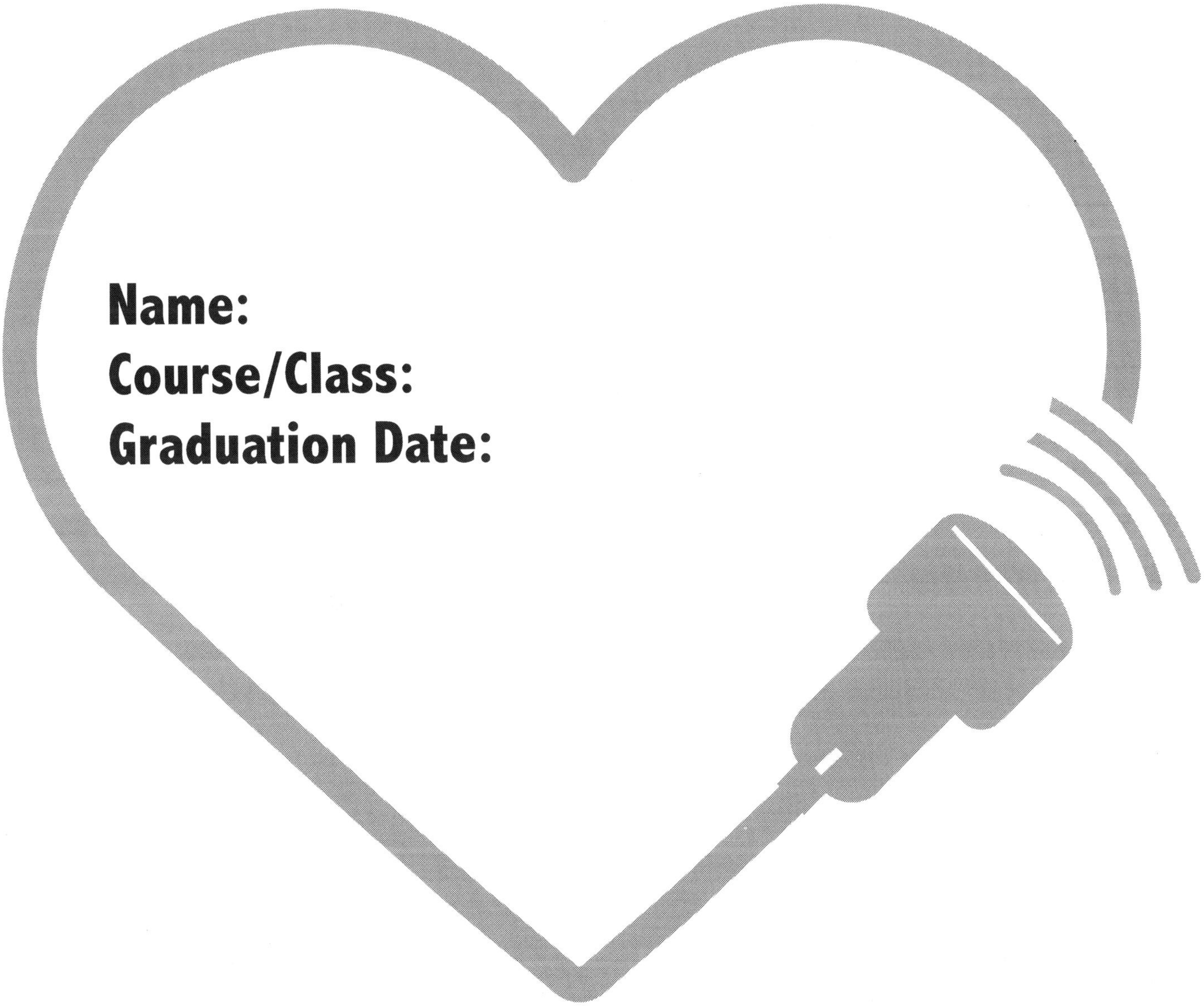

Name:
Course/Class:
Graduation Date:

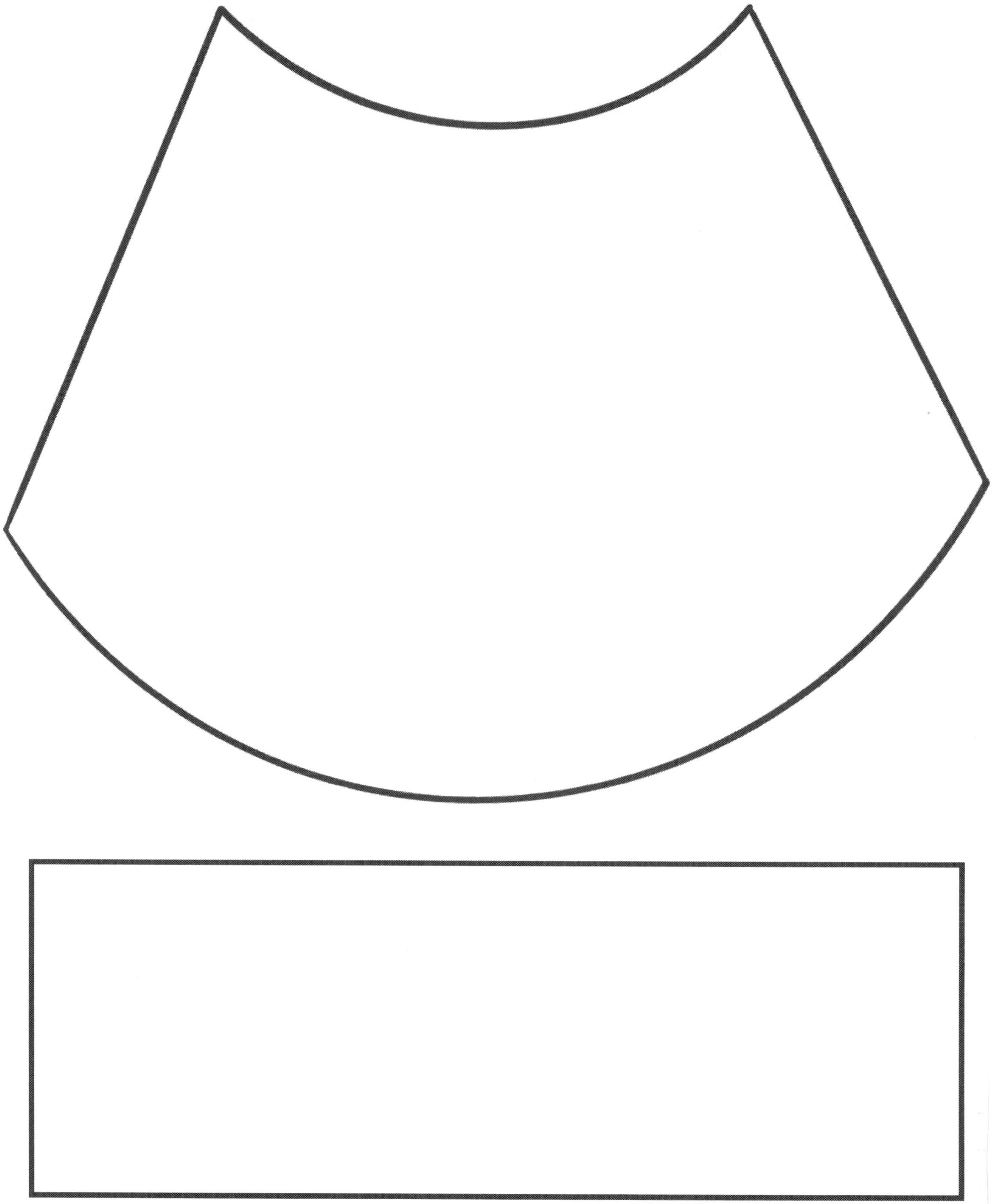

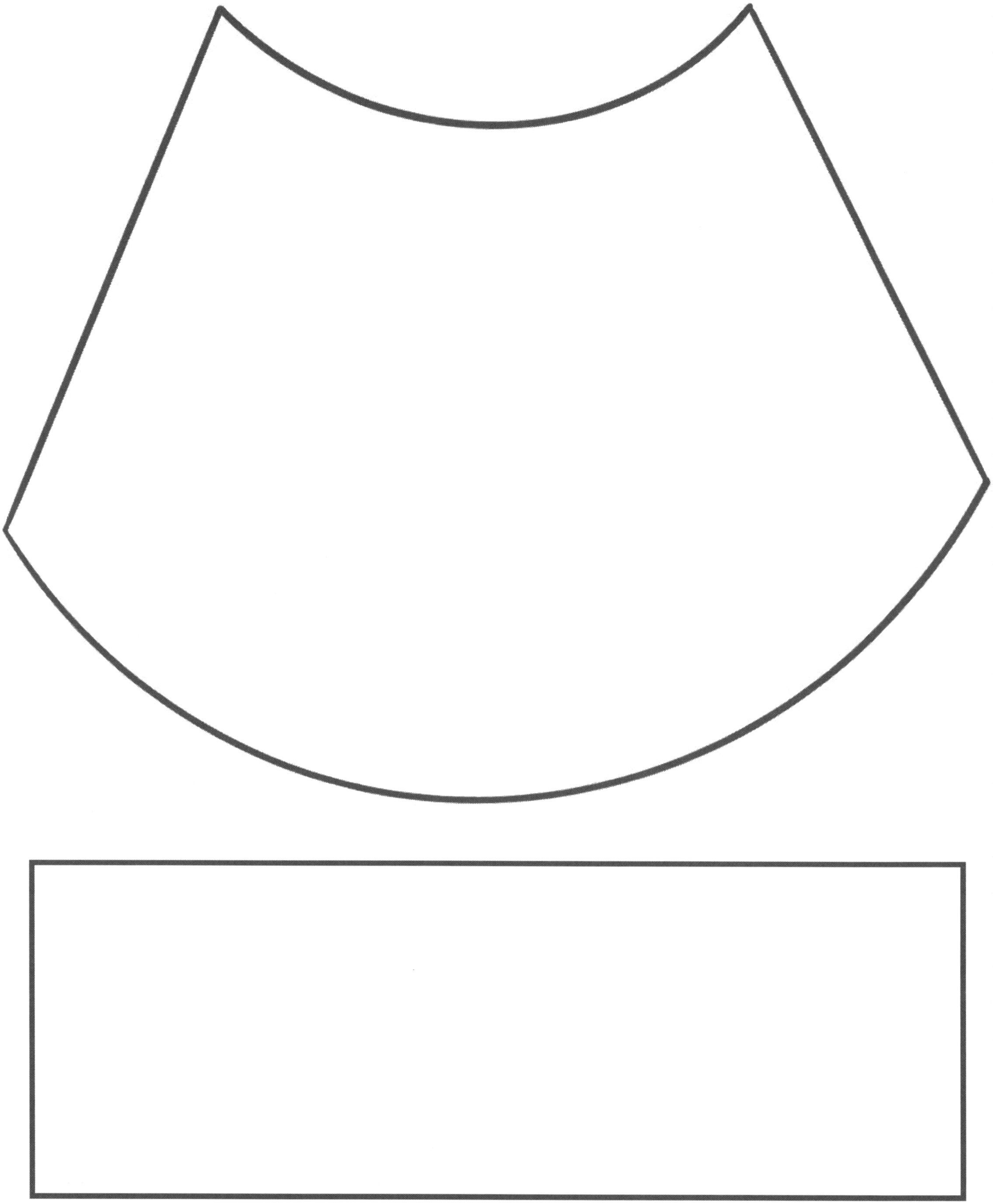

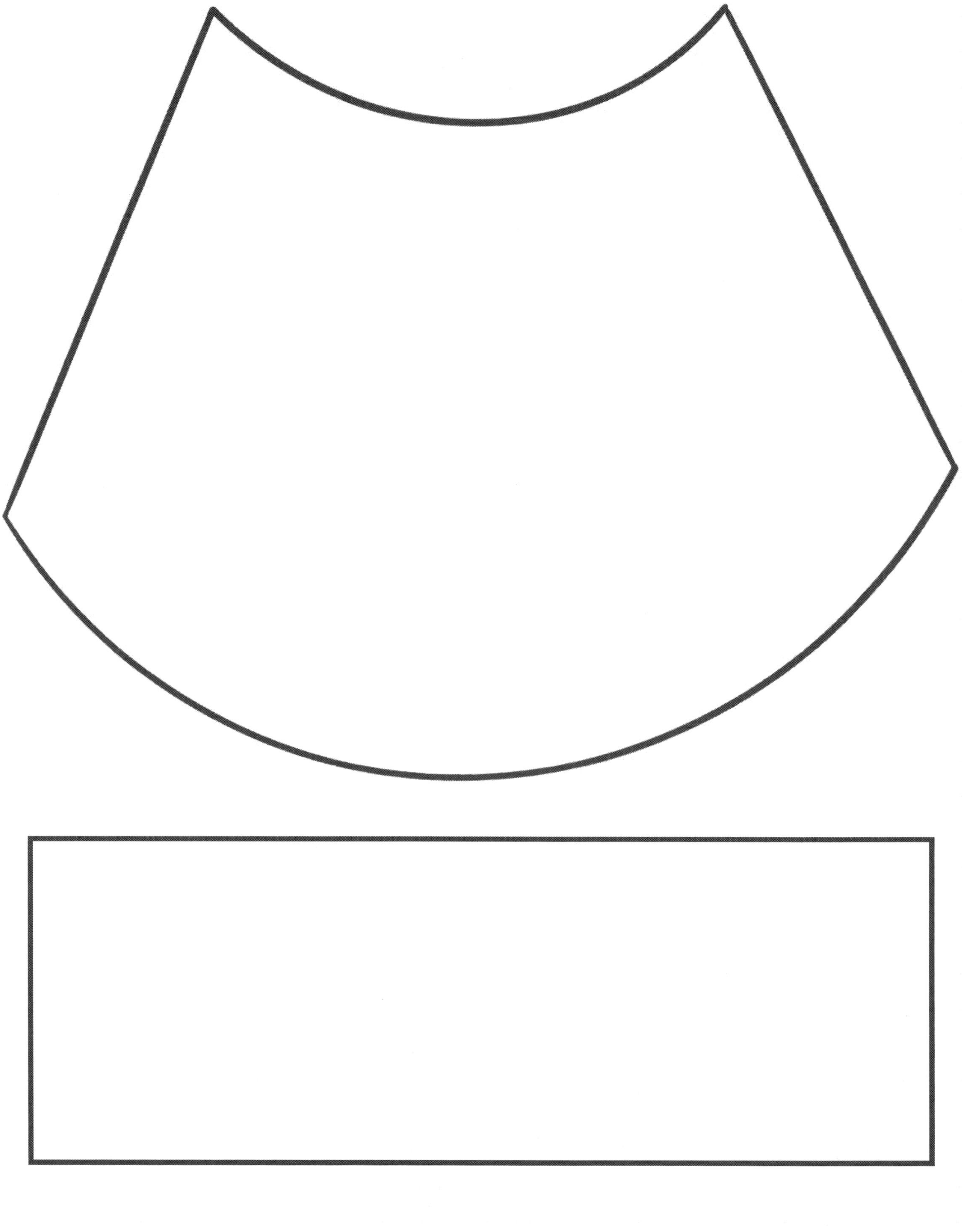

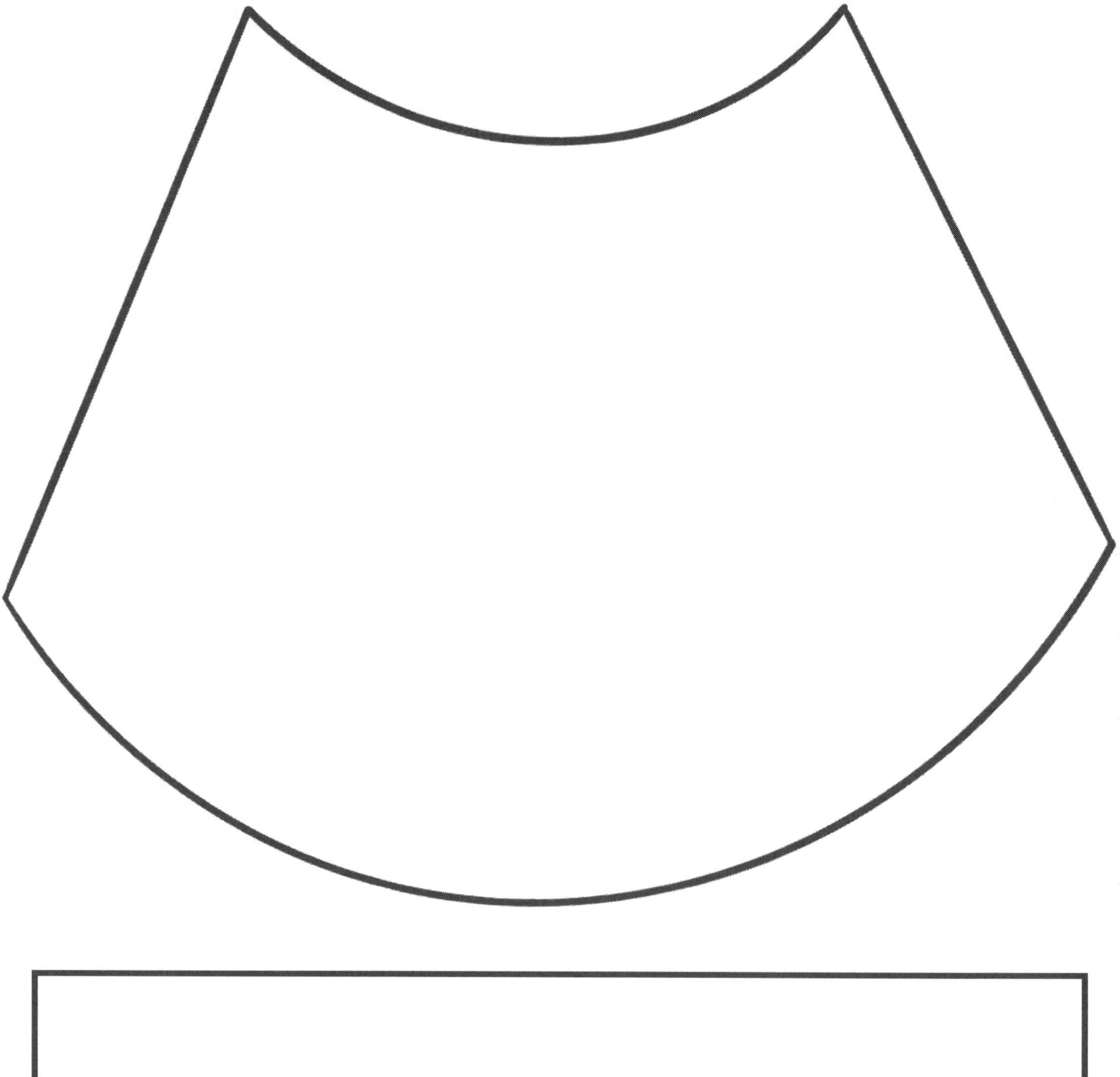

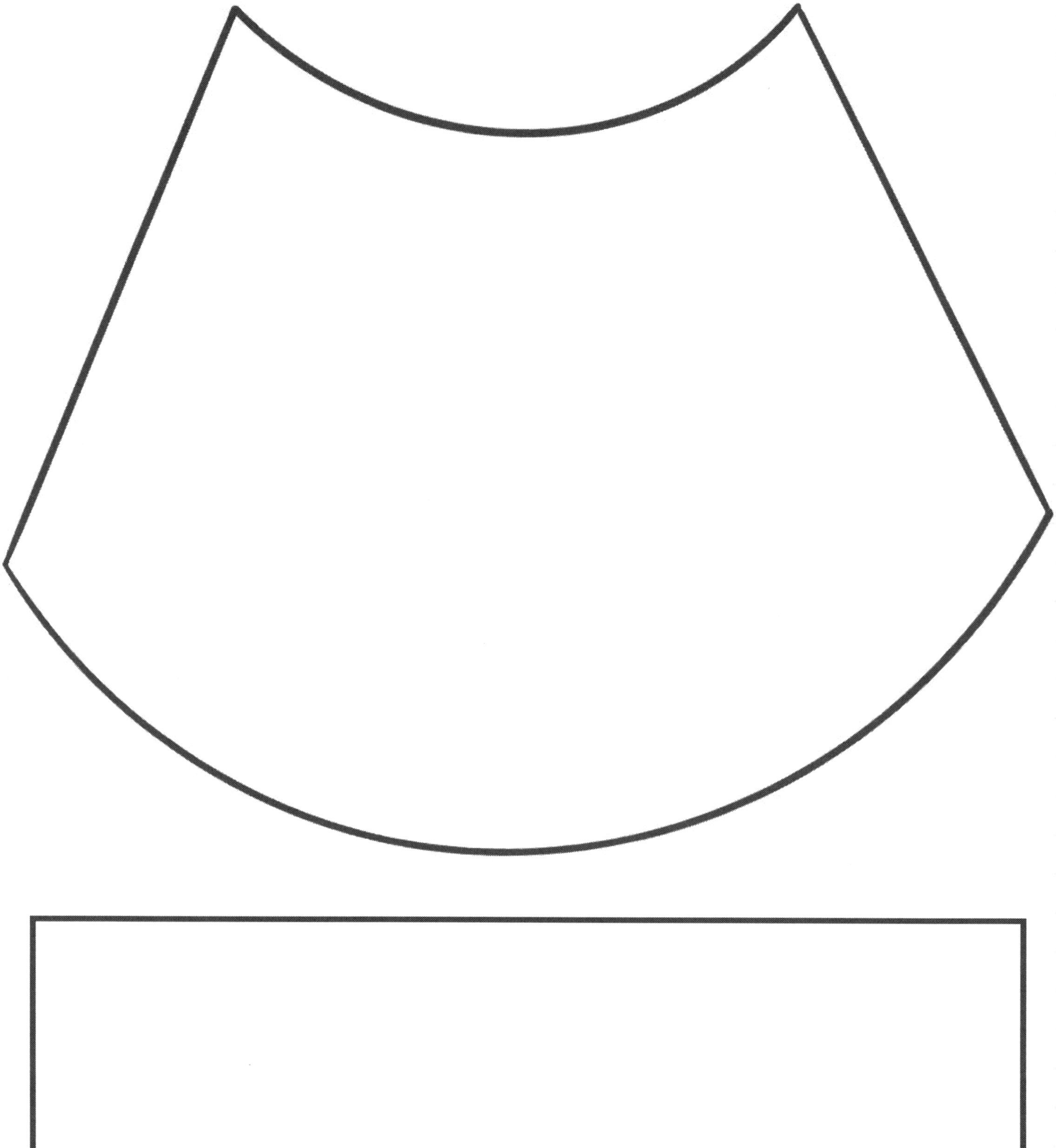

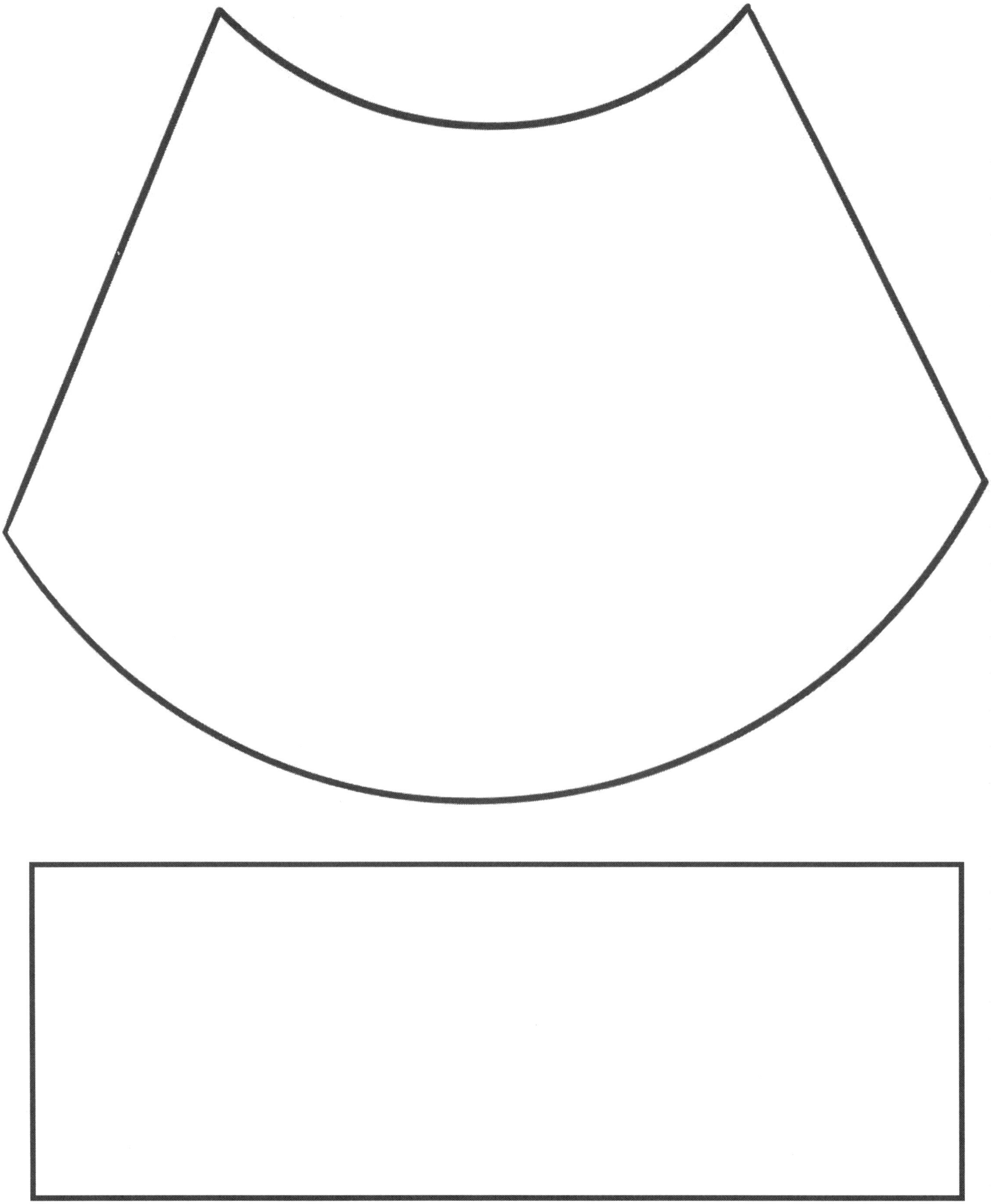

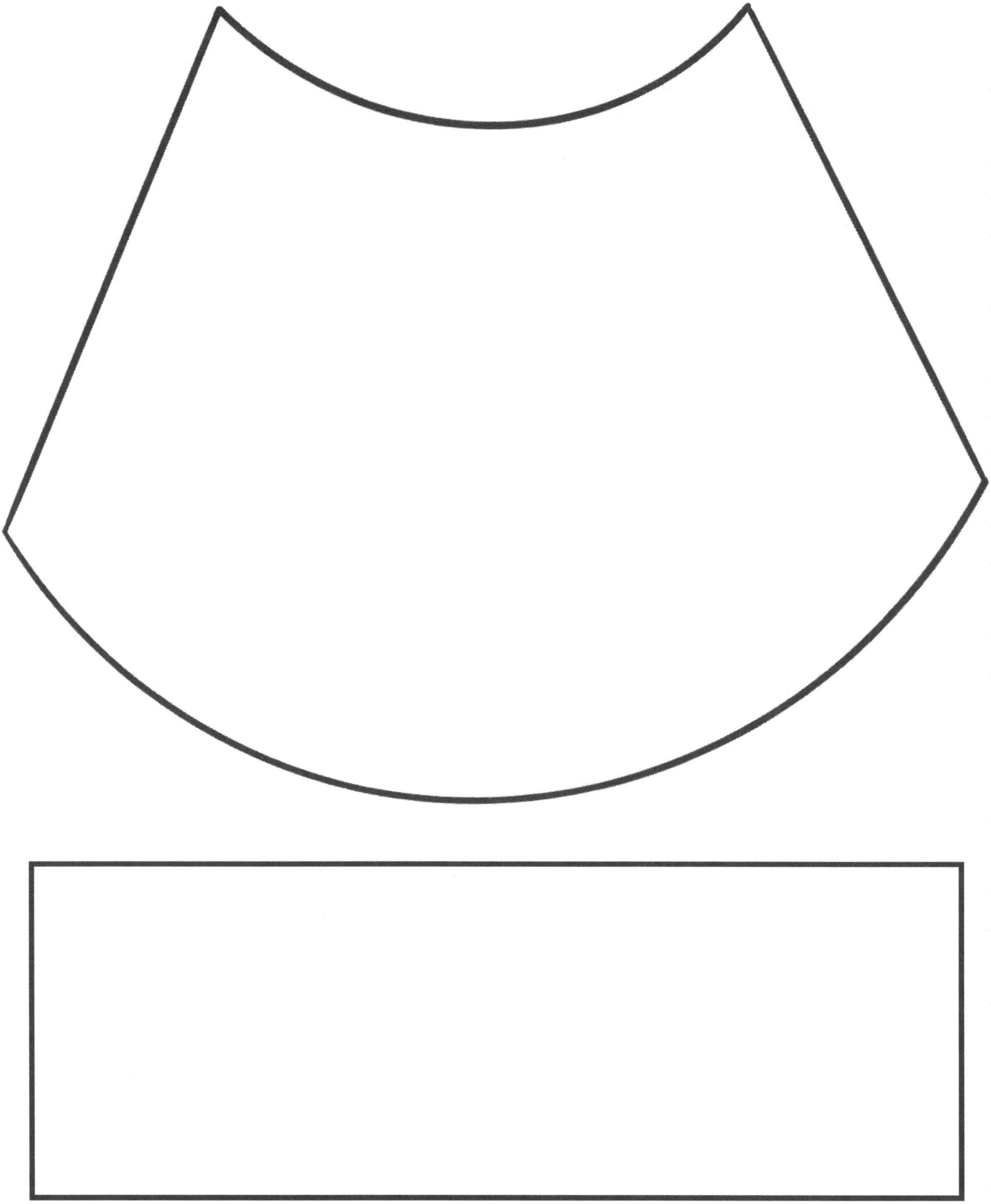

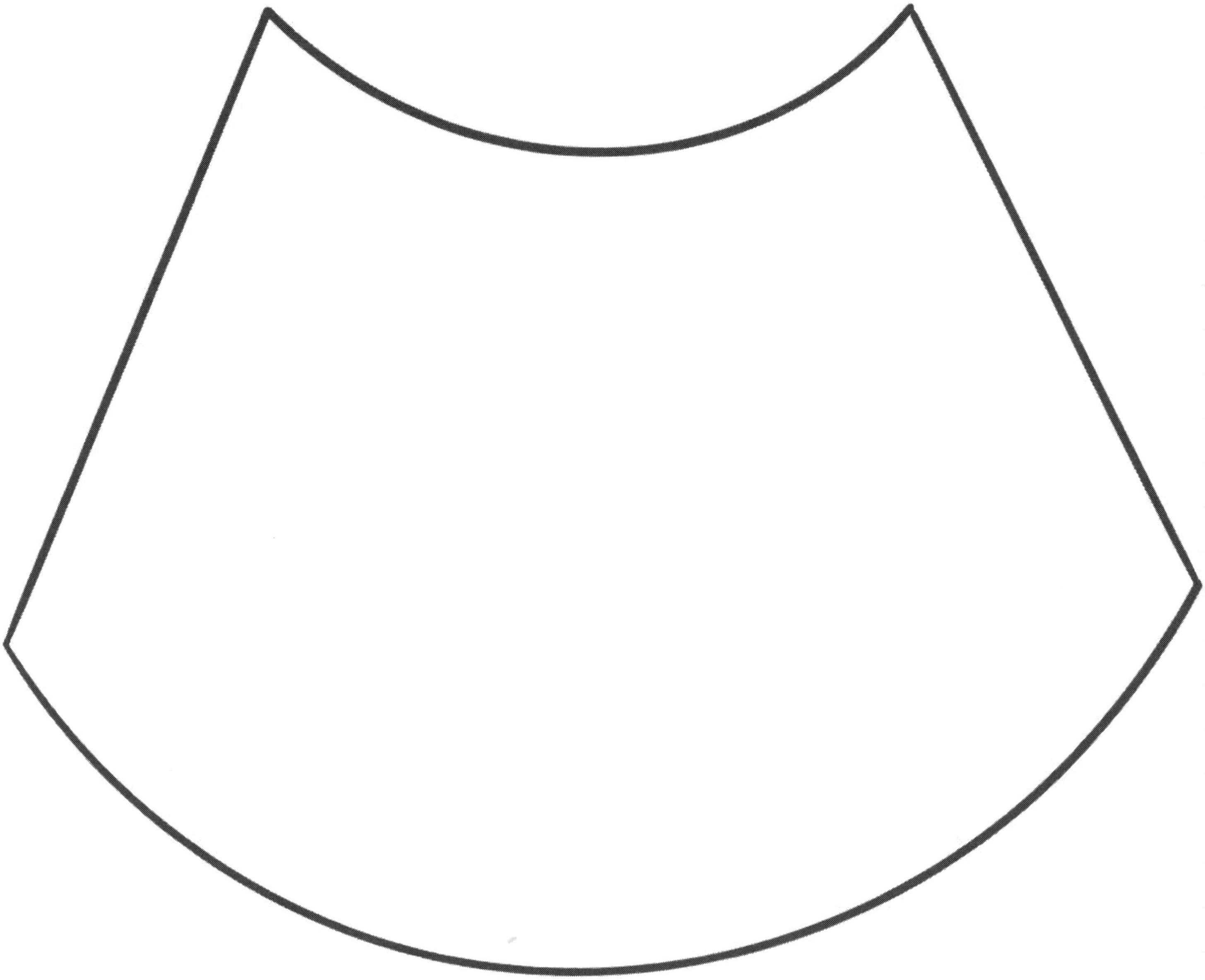

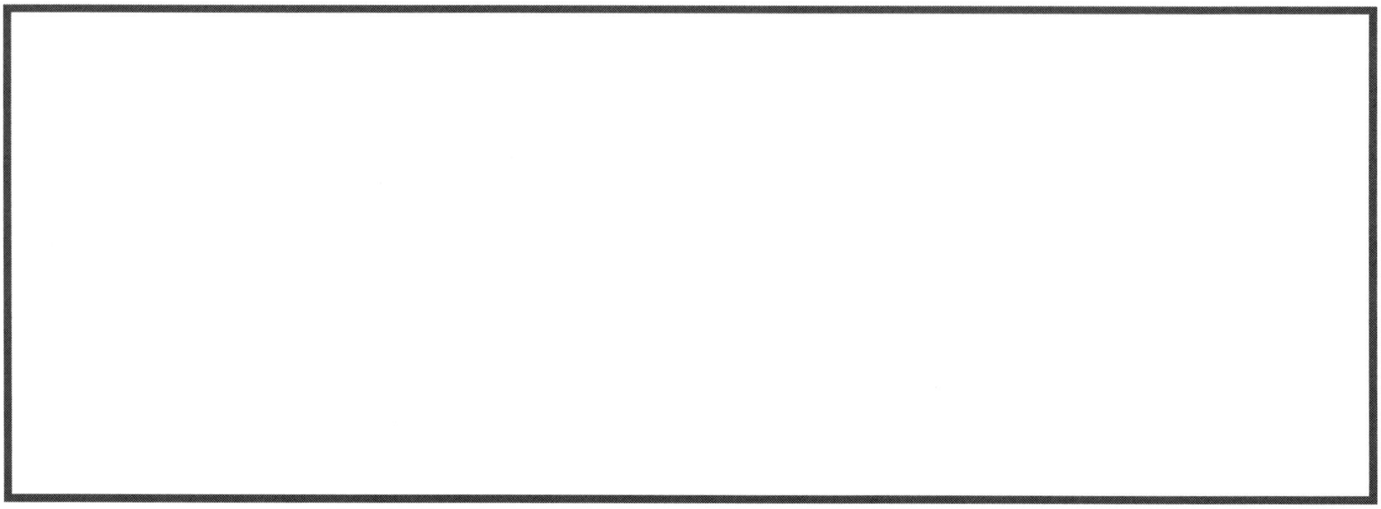

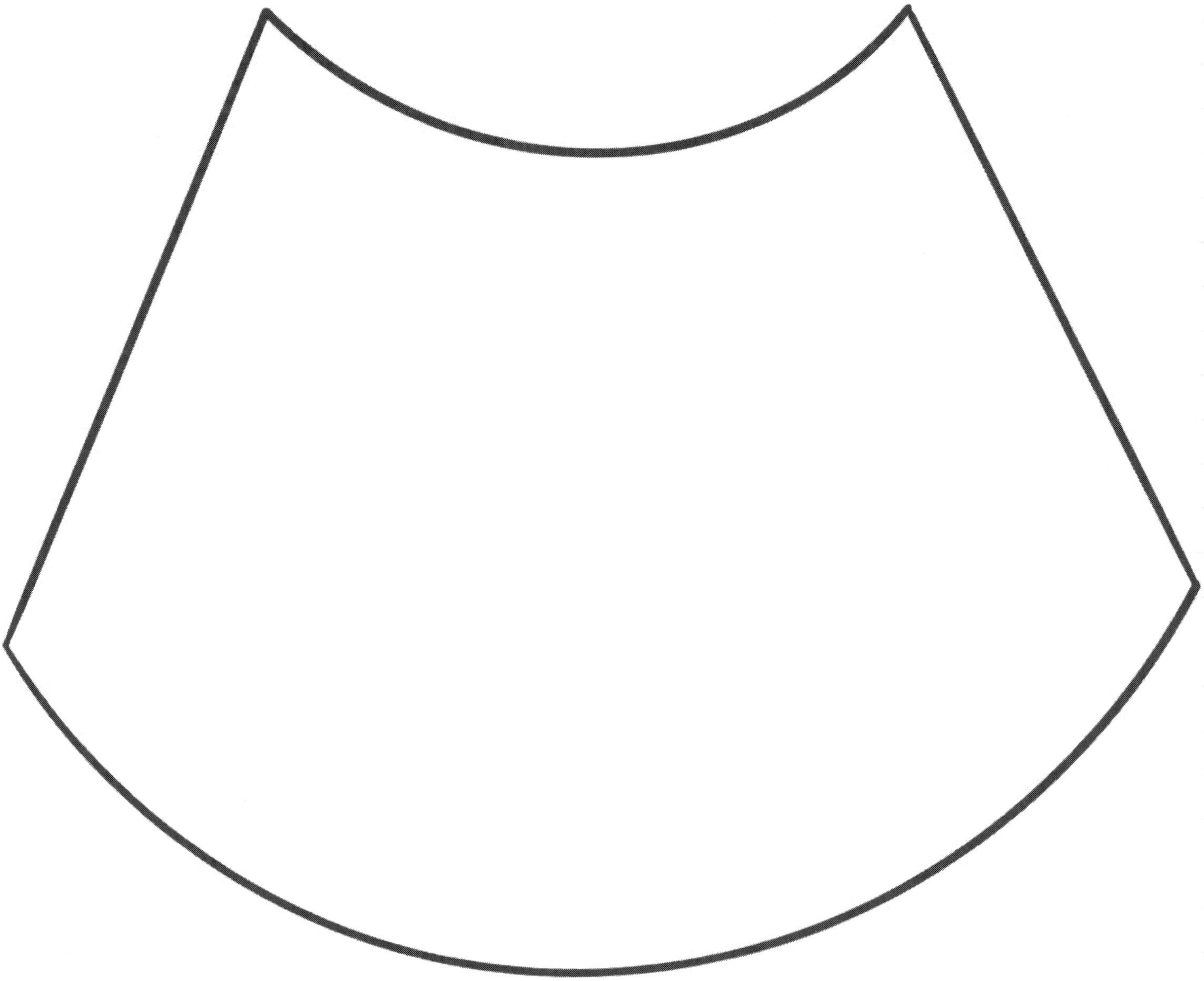
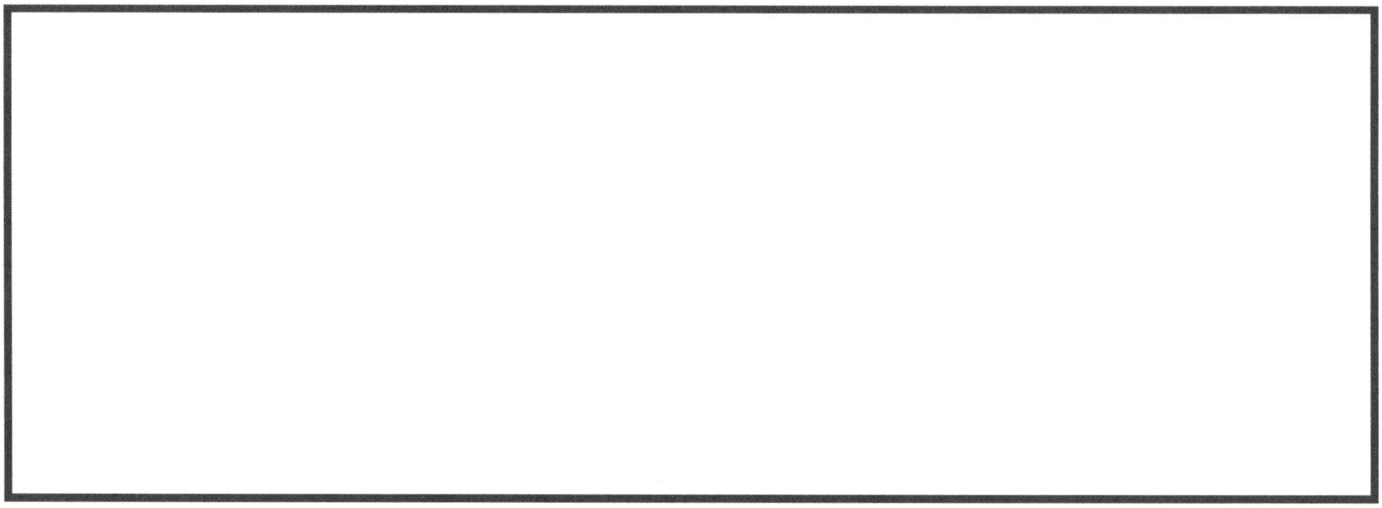

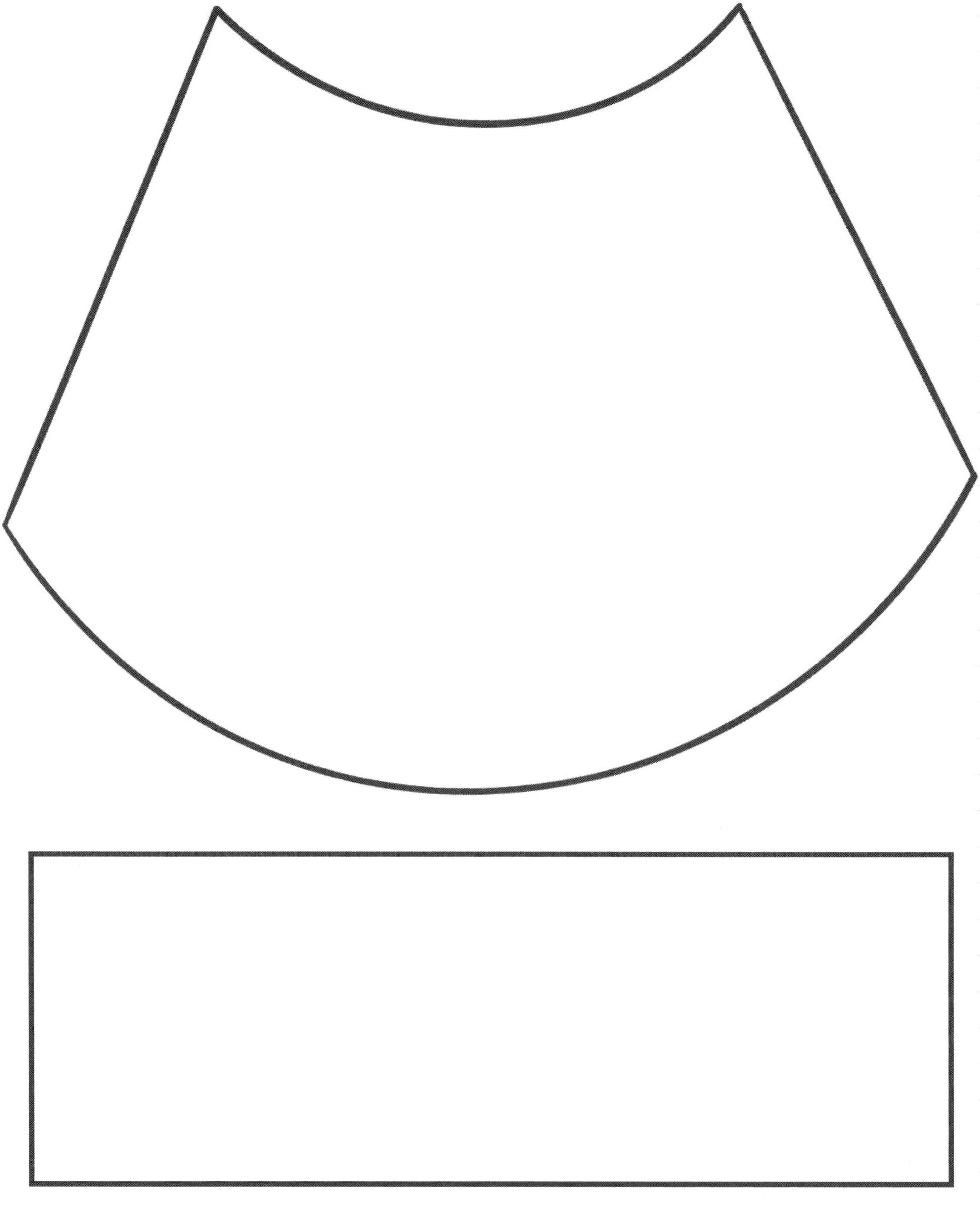

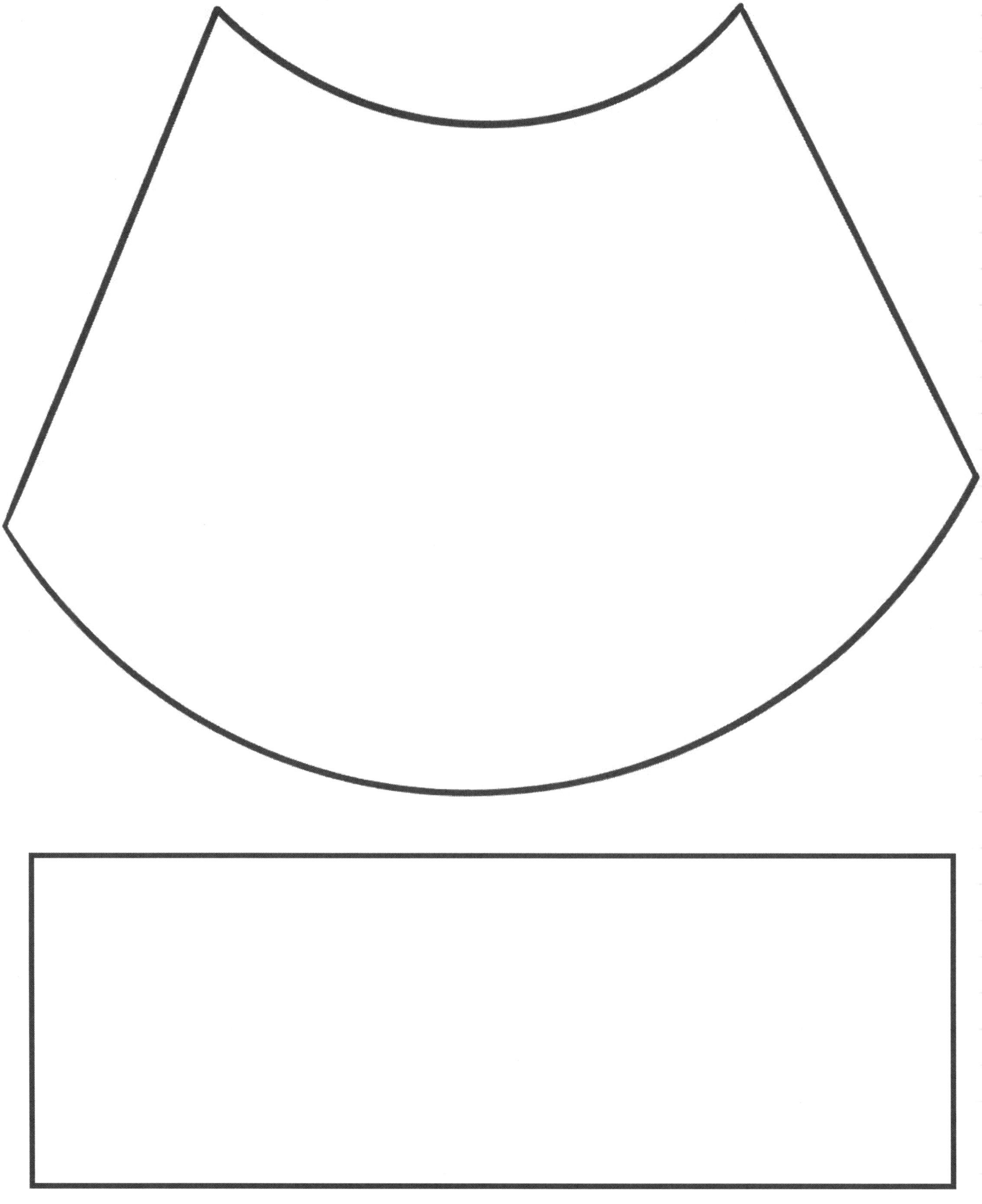

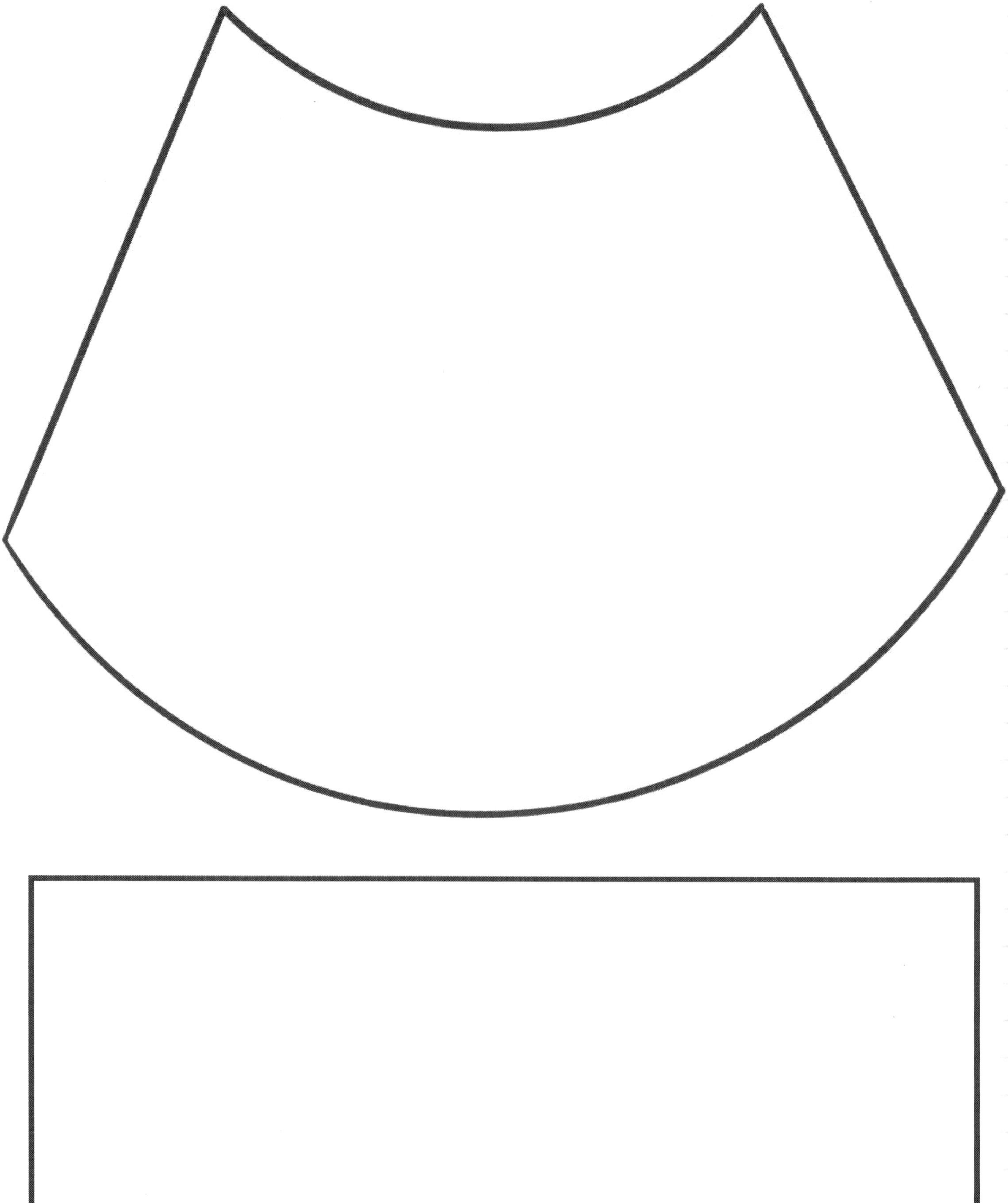

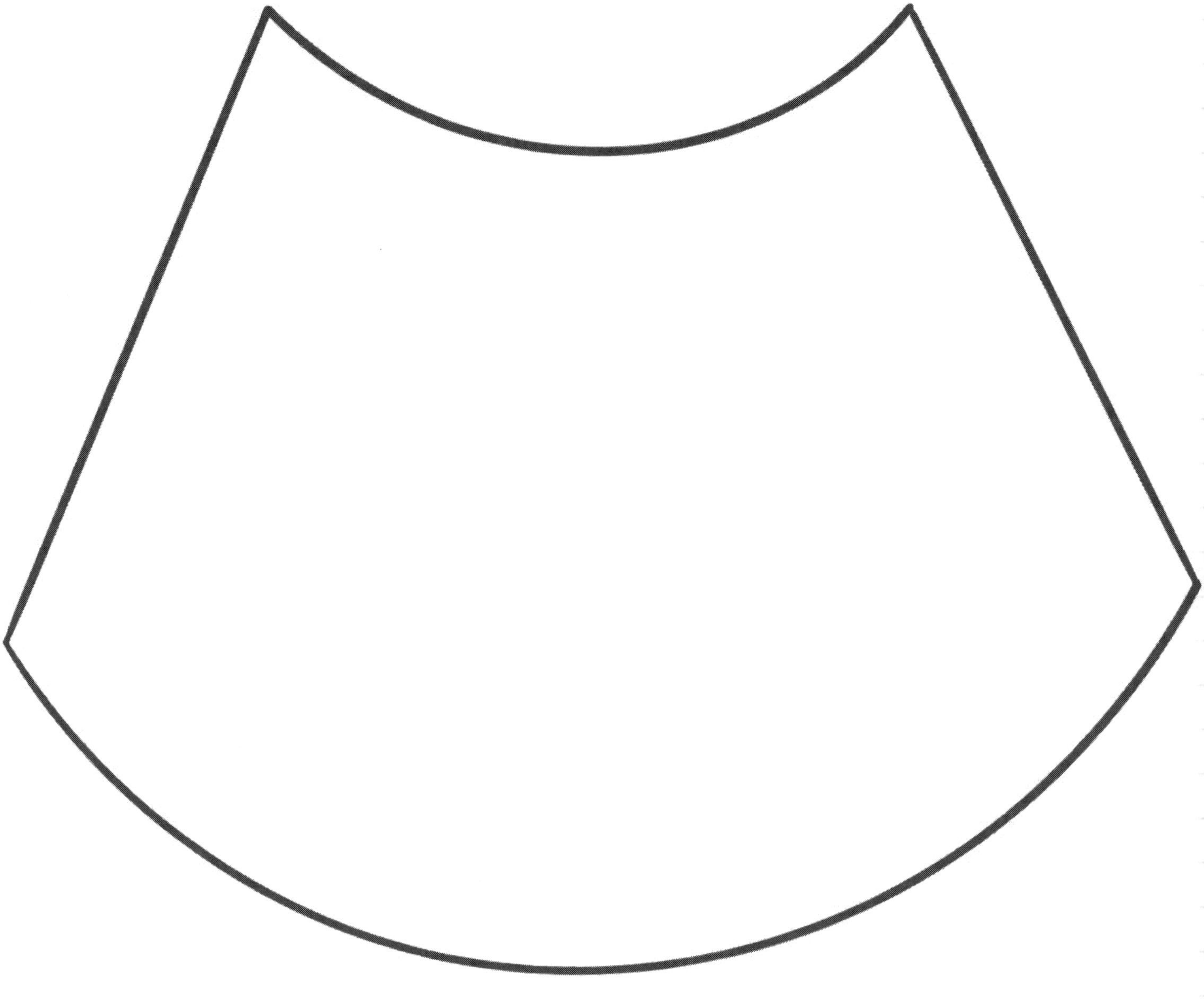

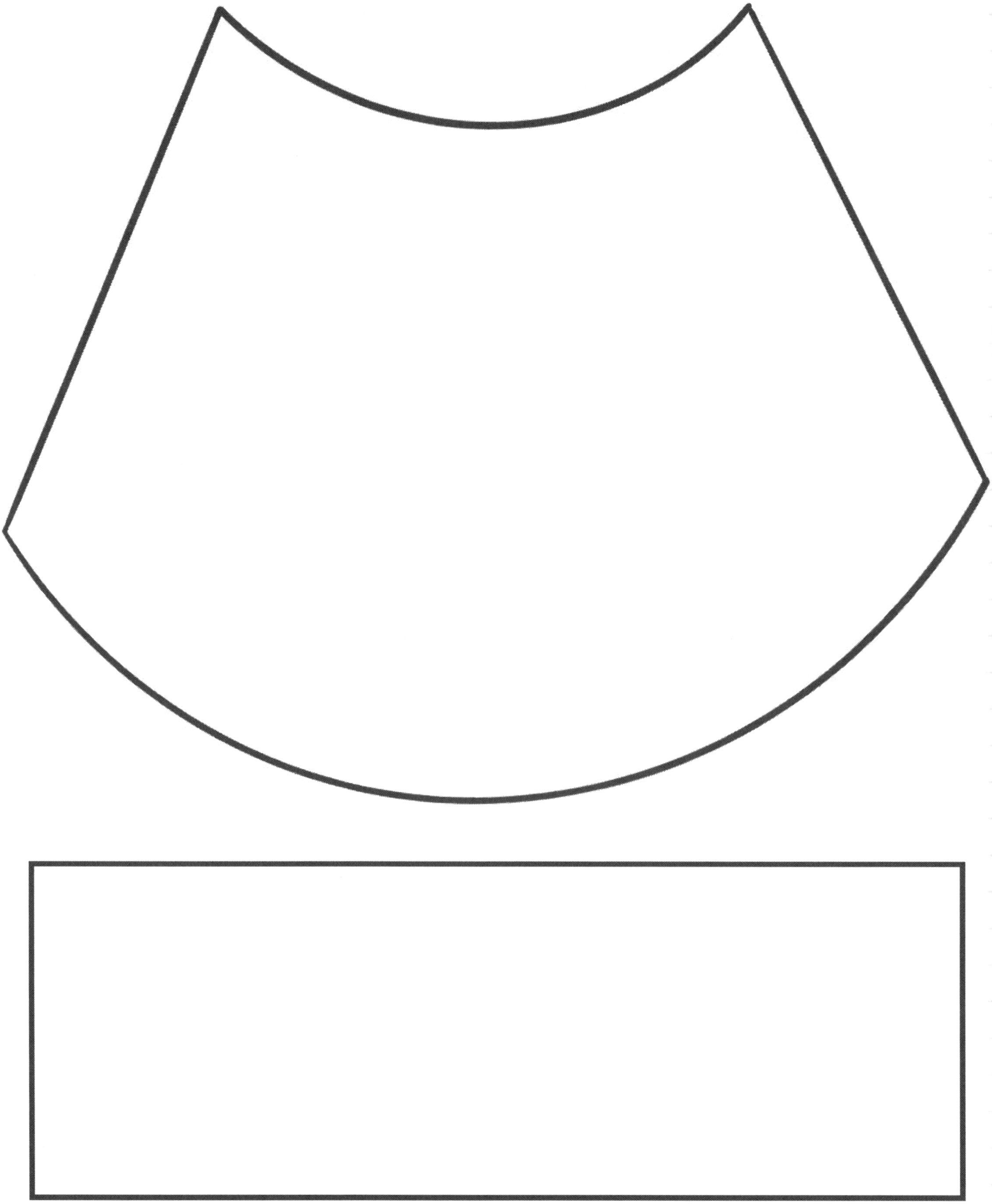

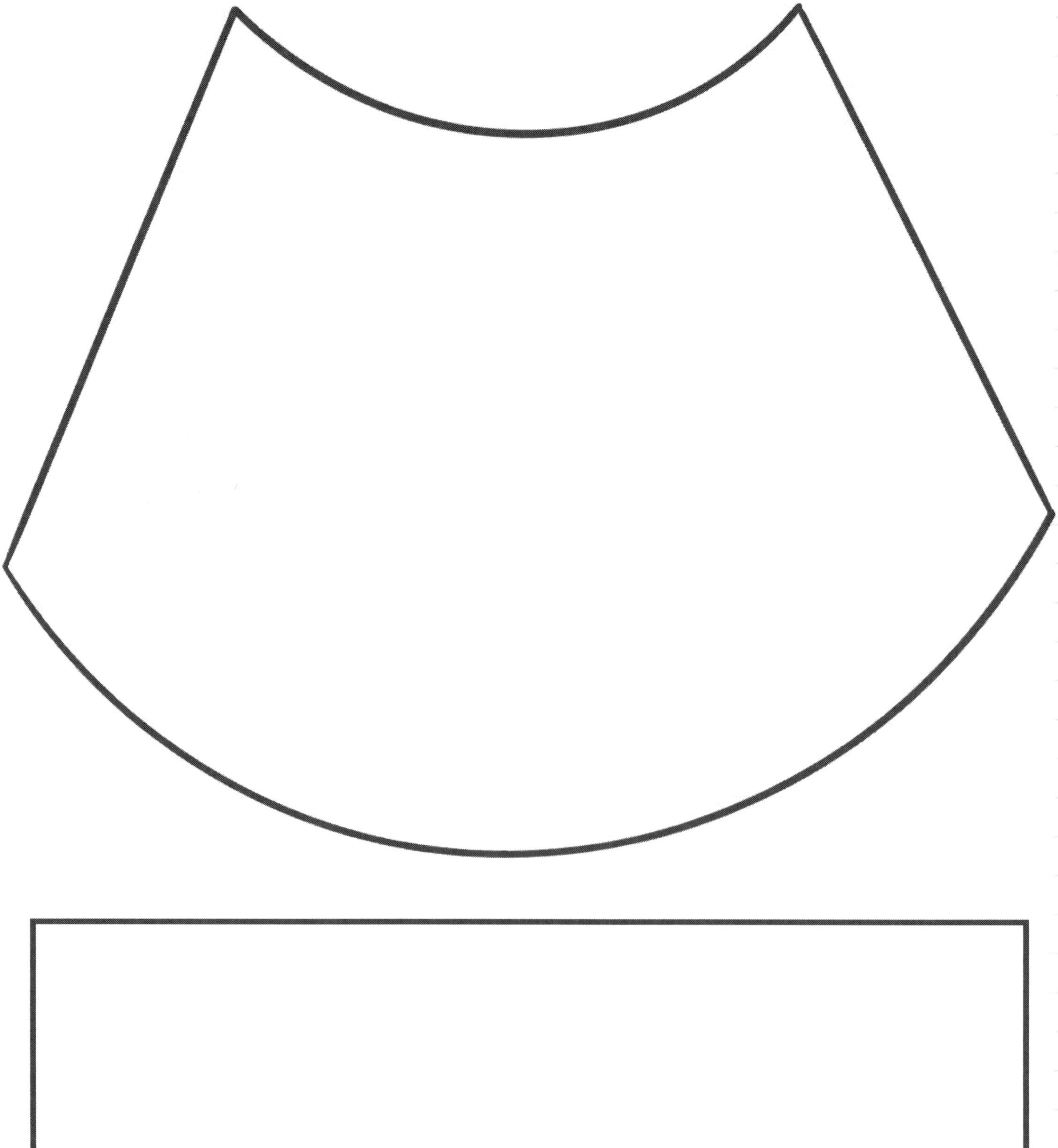

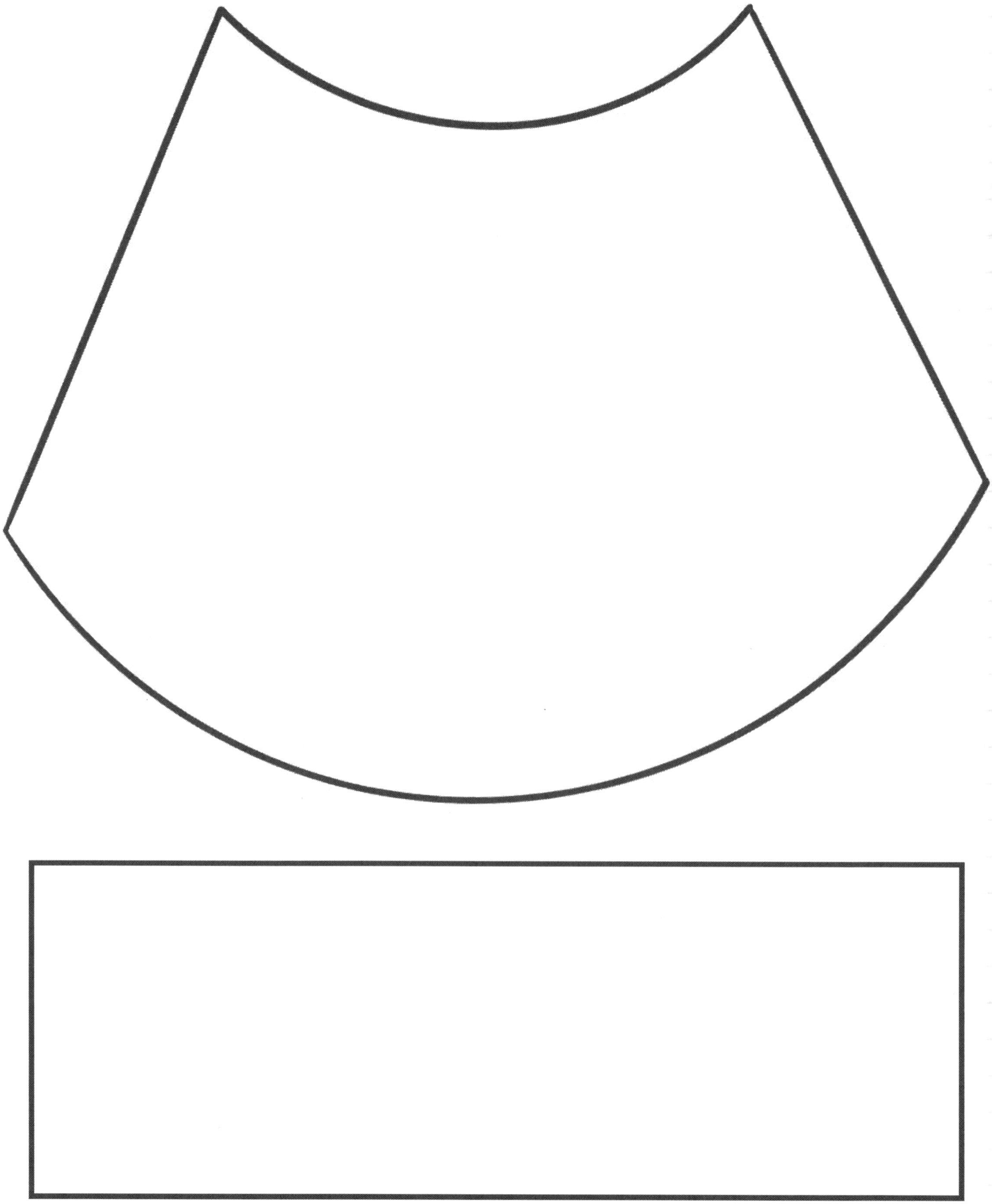

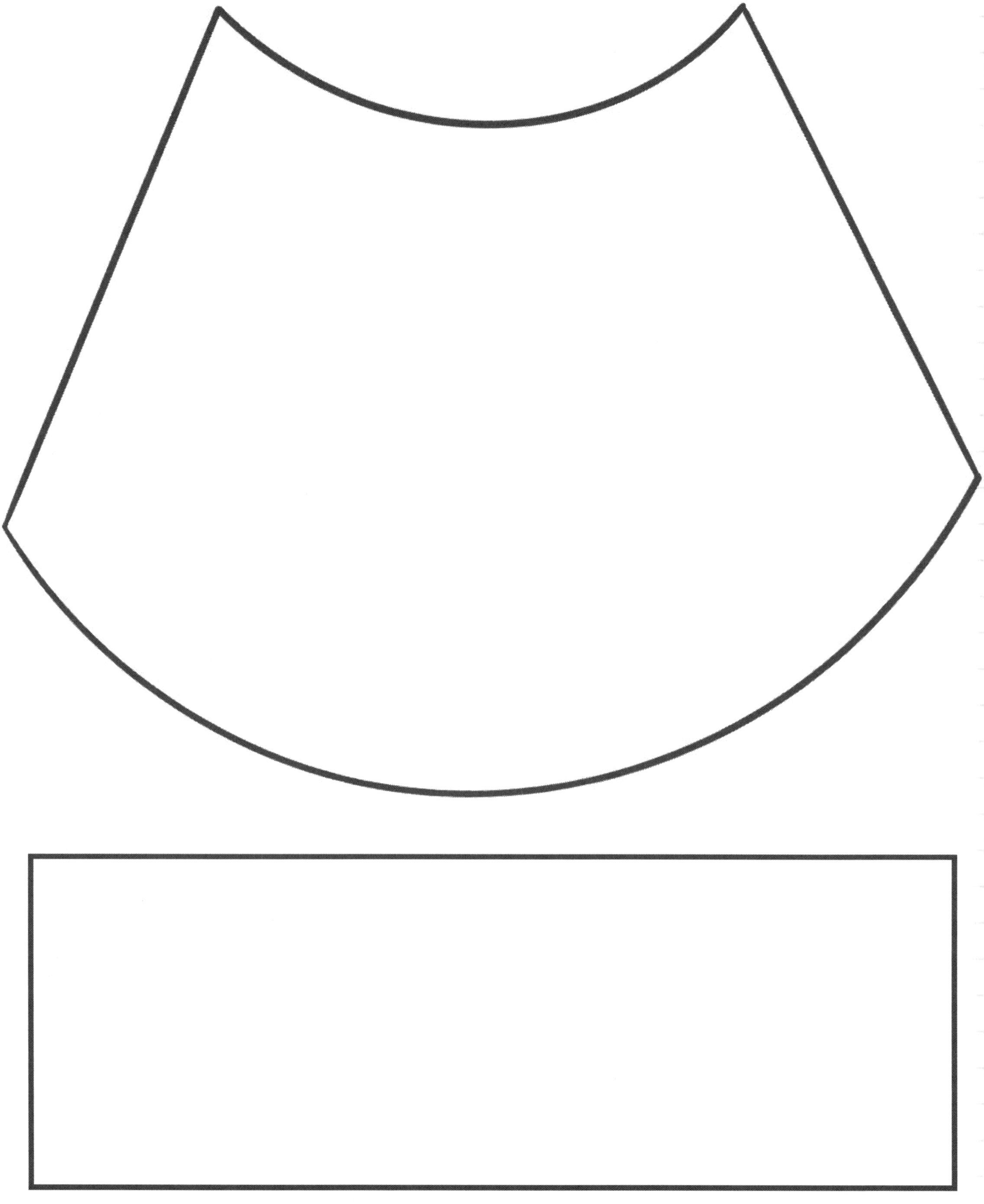

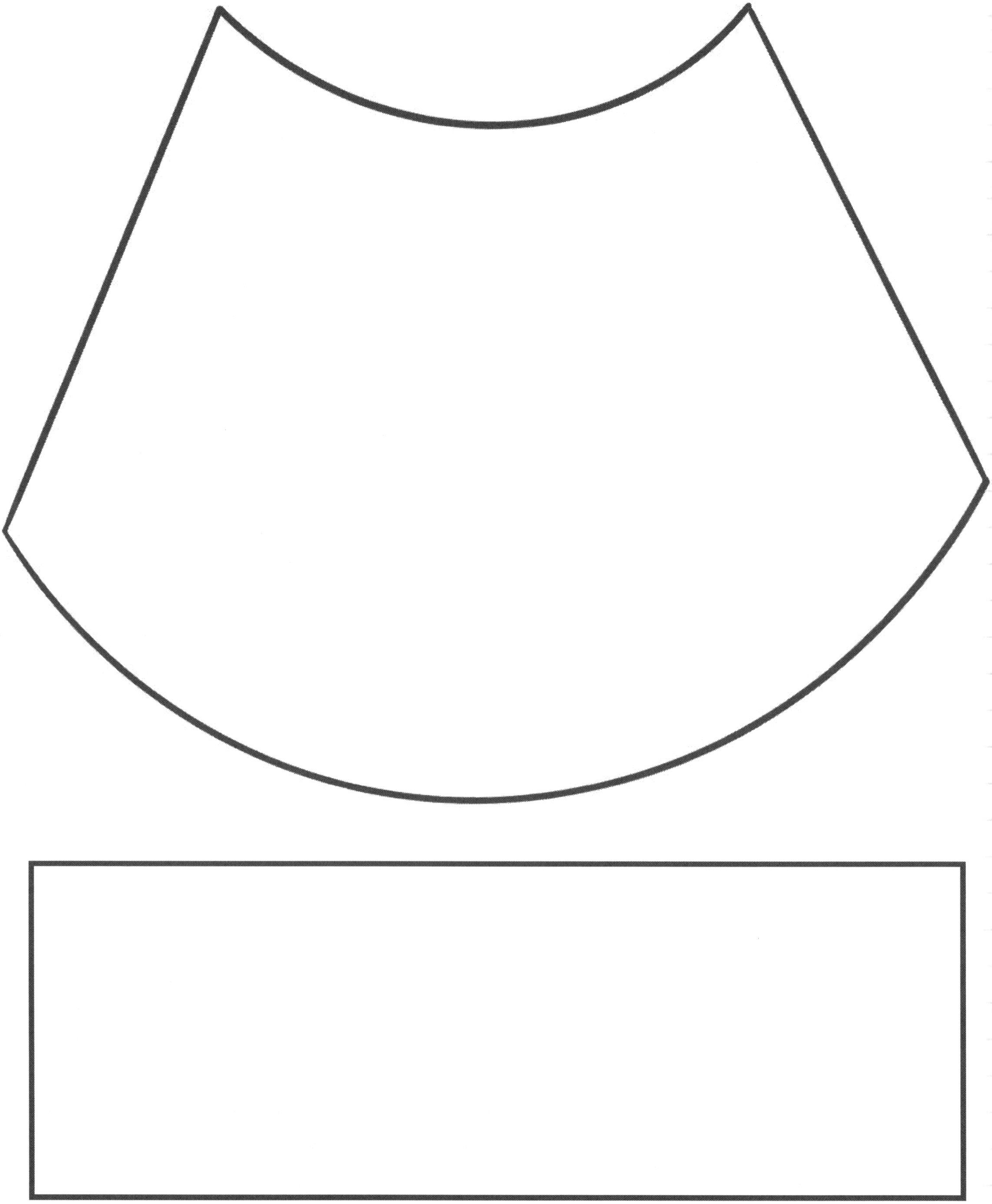

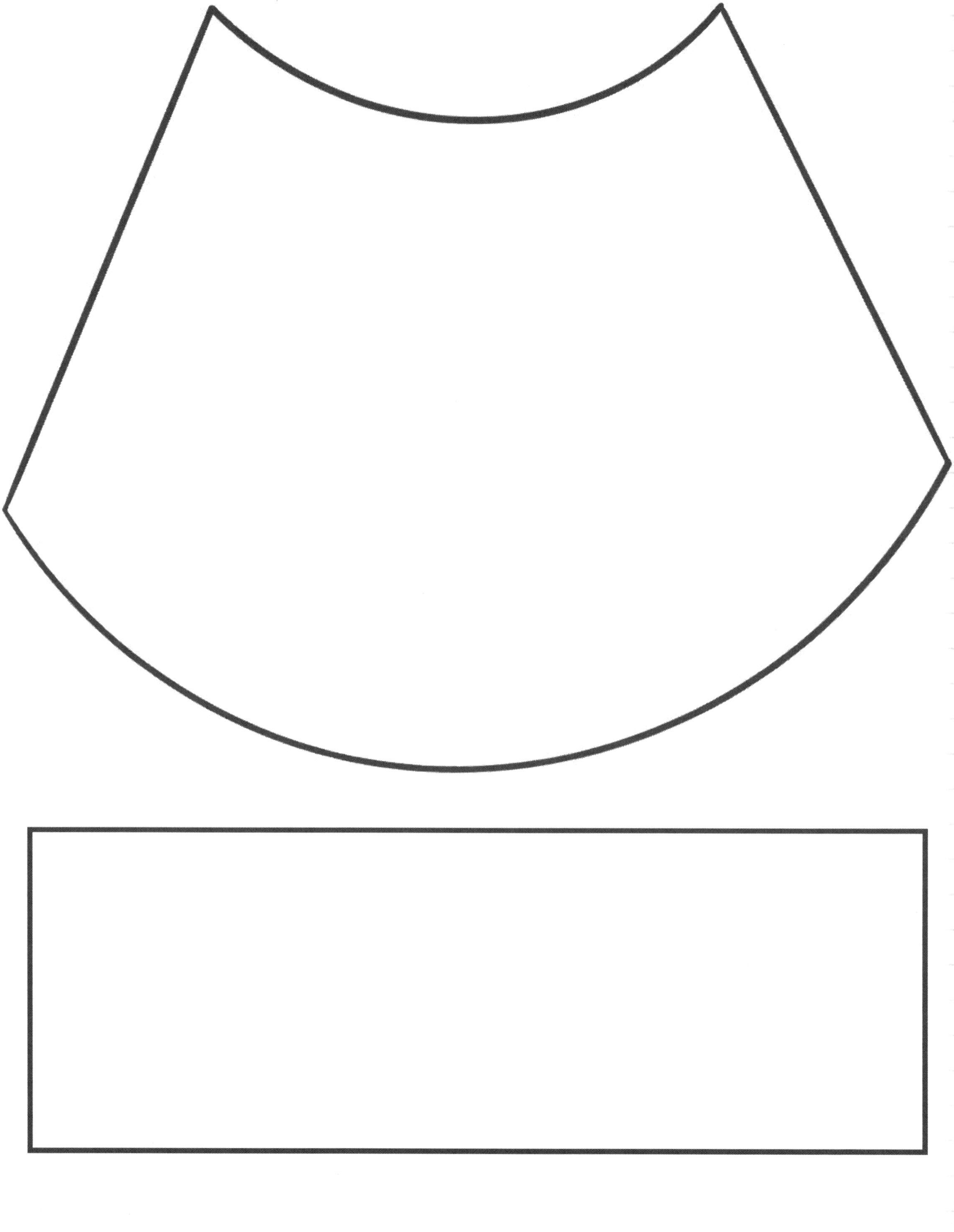

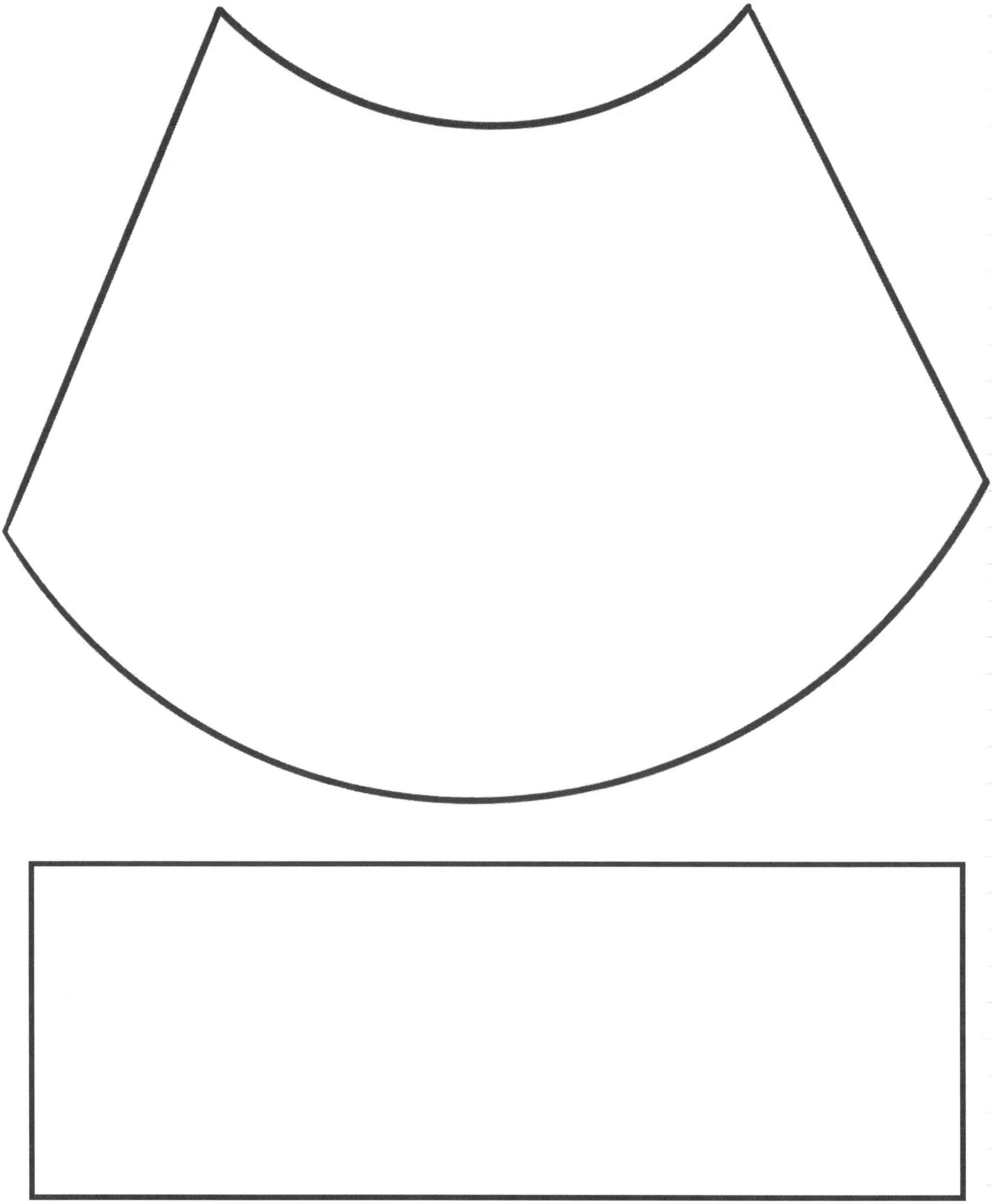

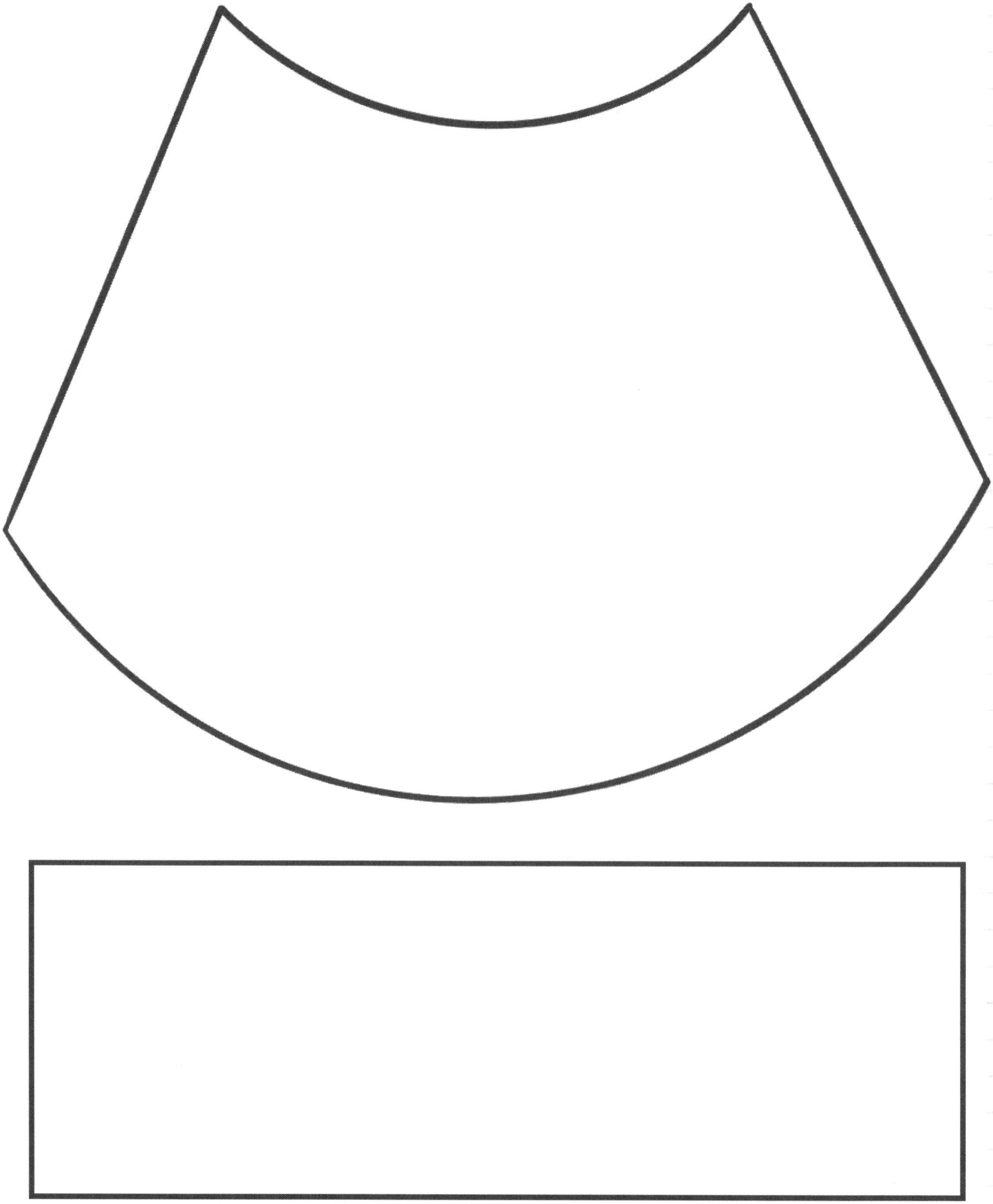

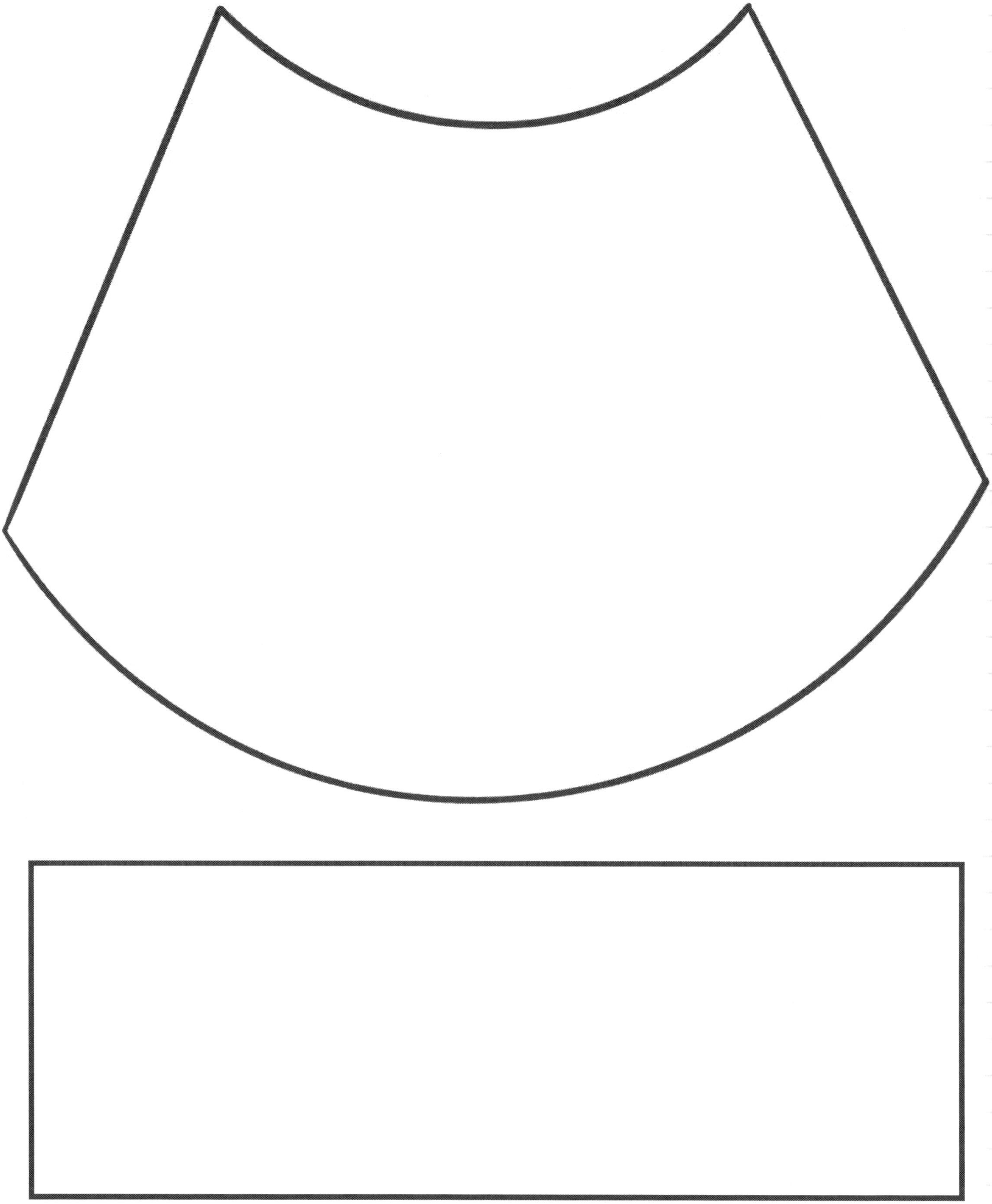

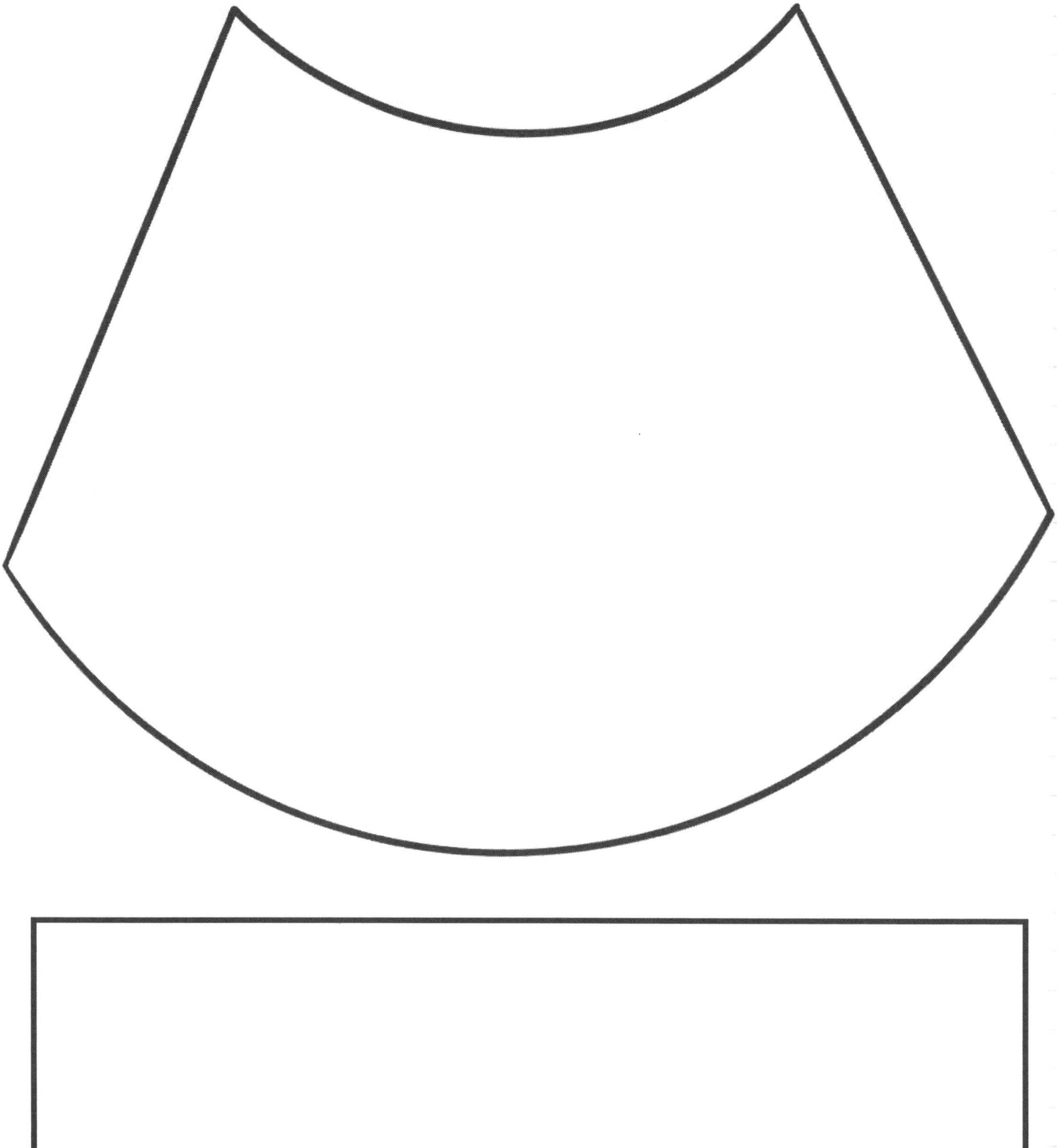

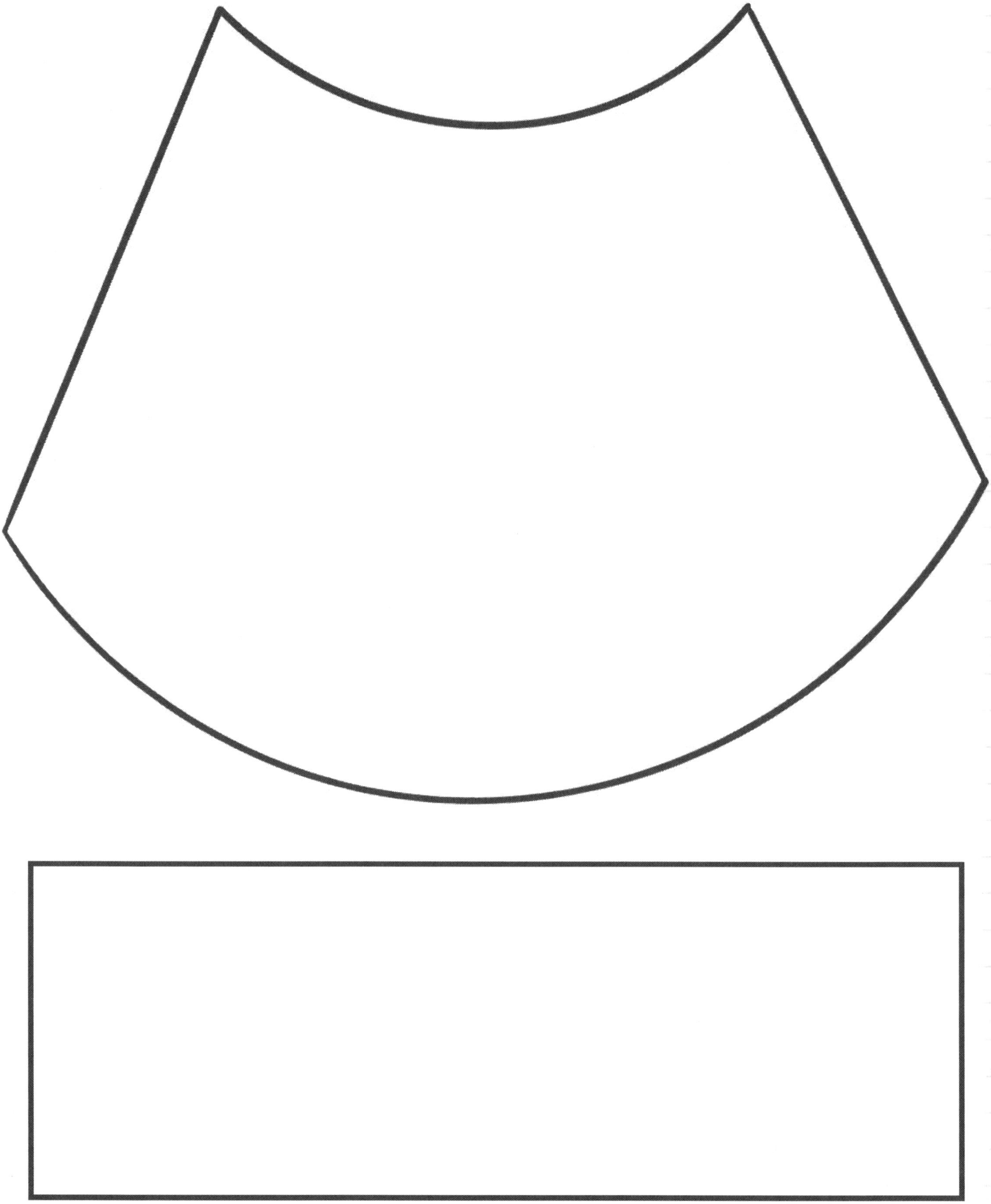

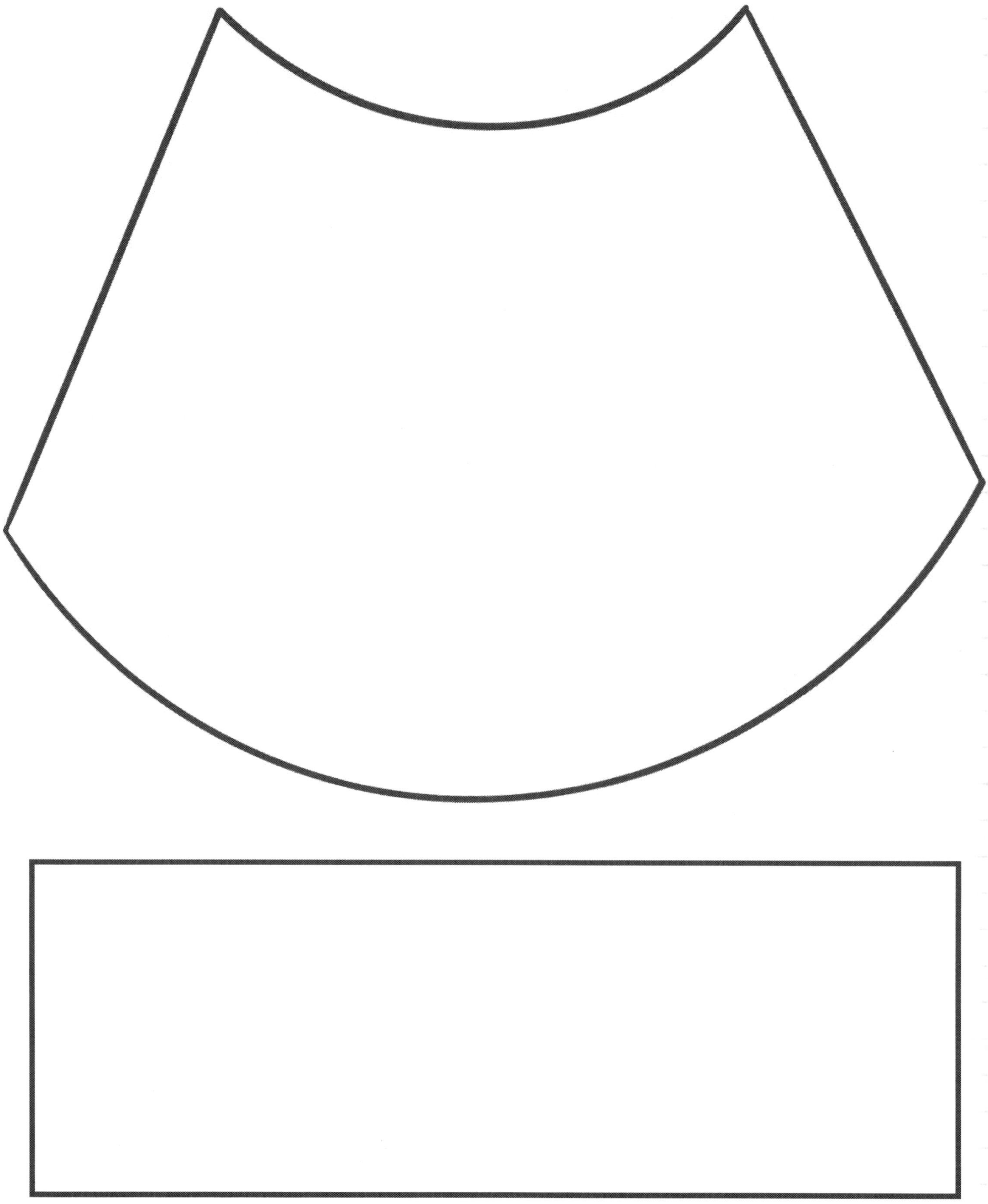

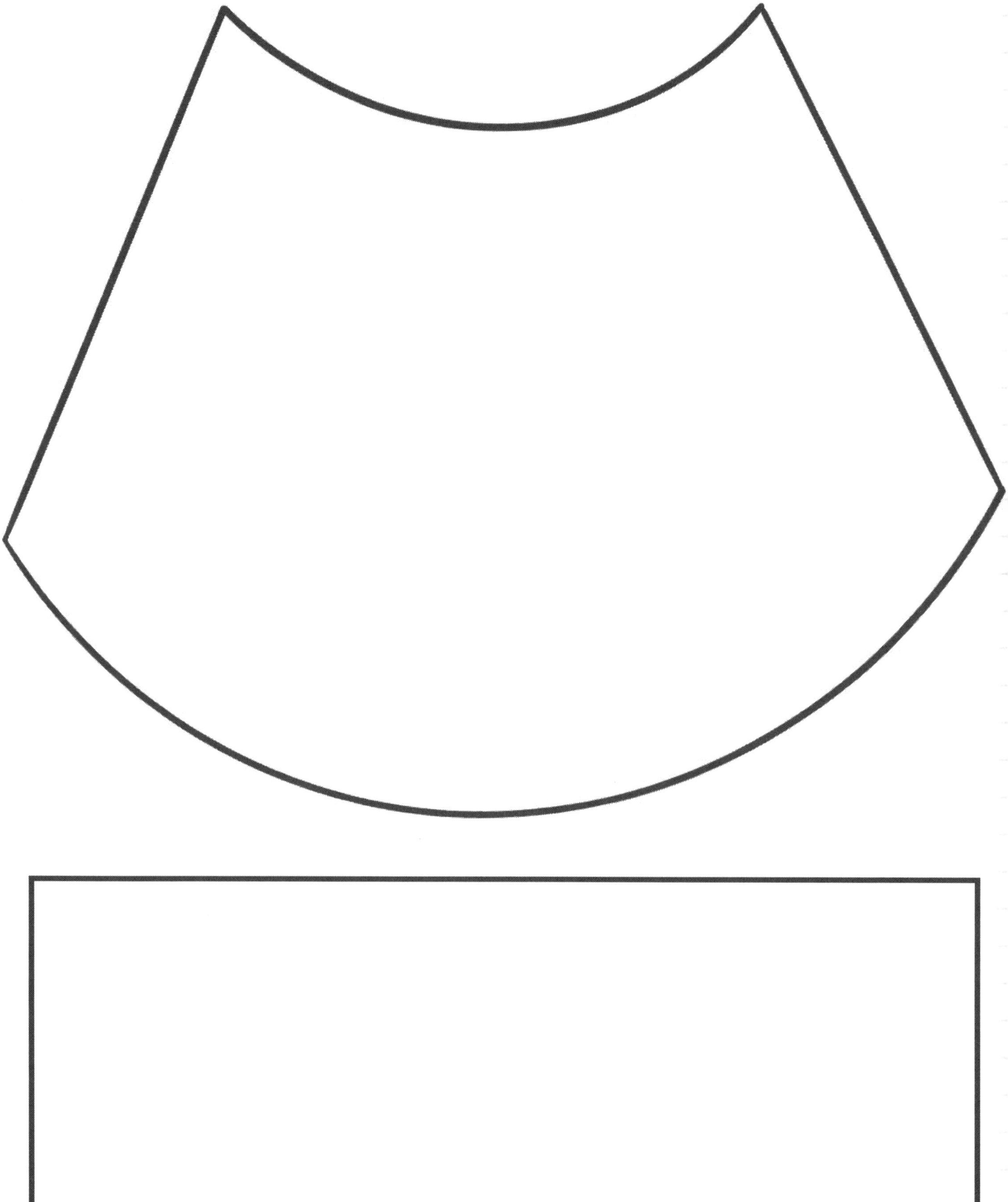

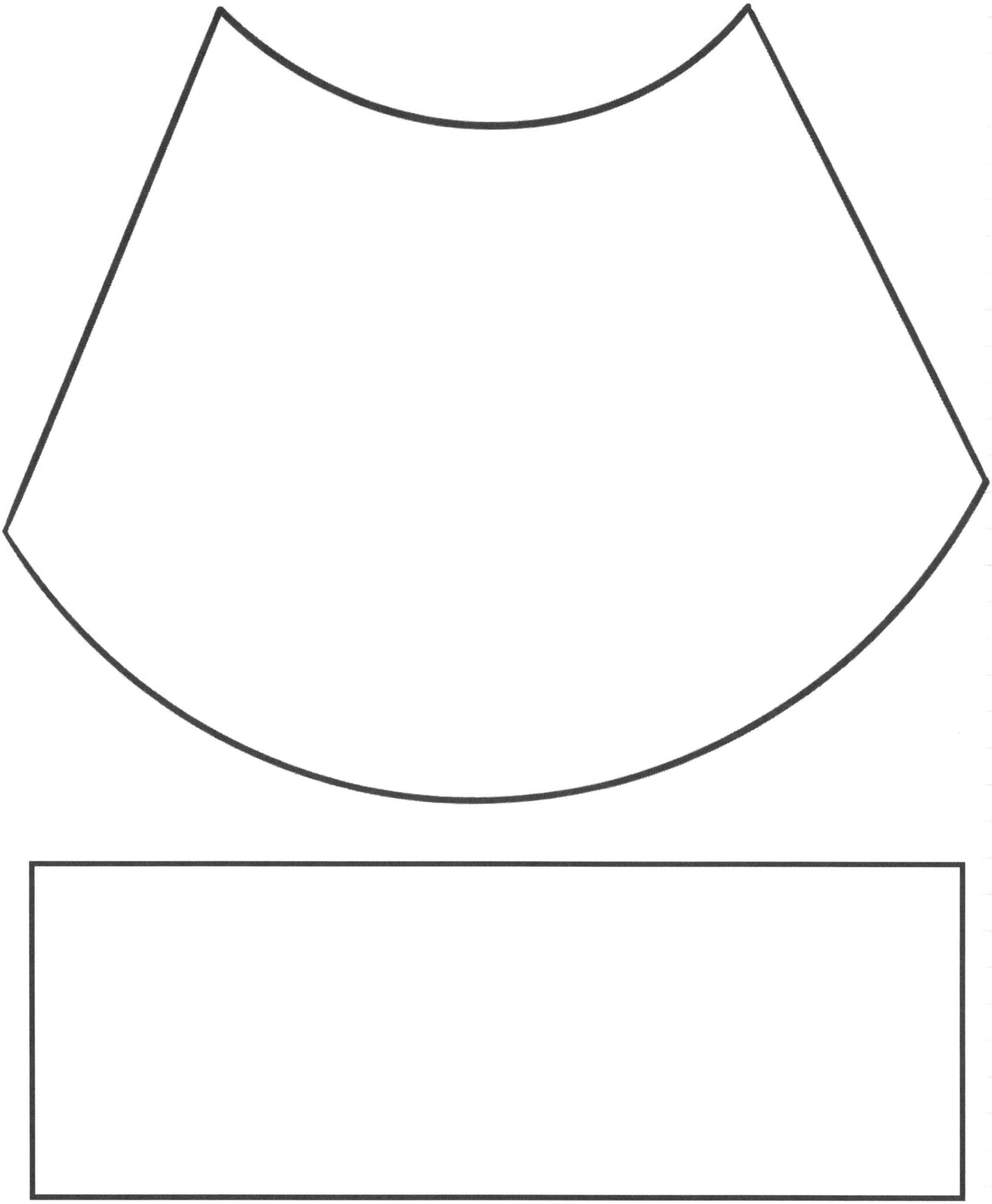

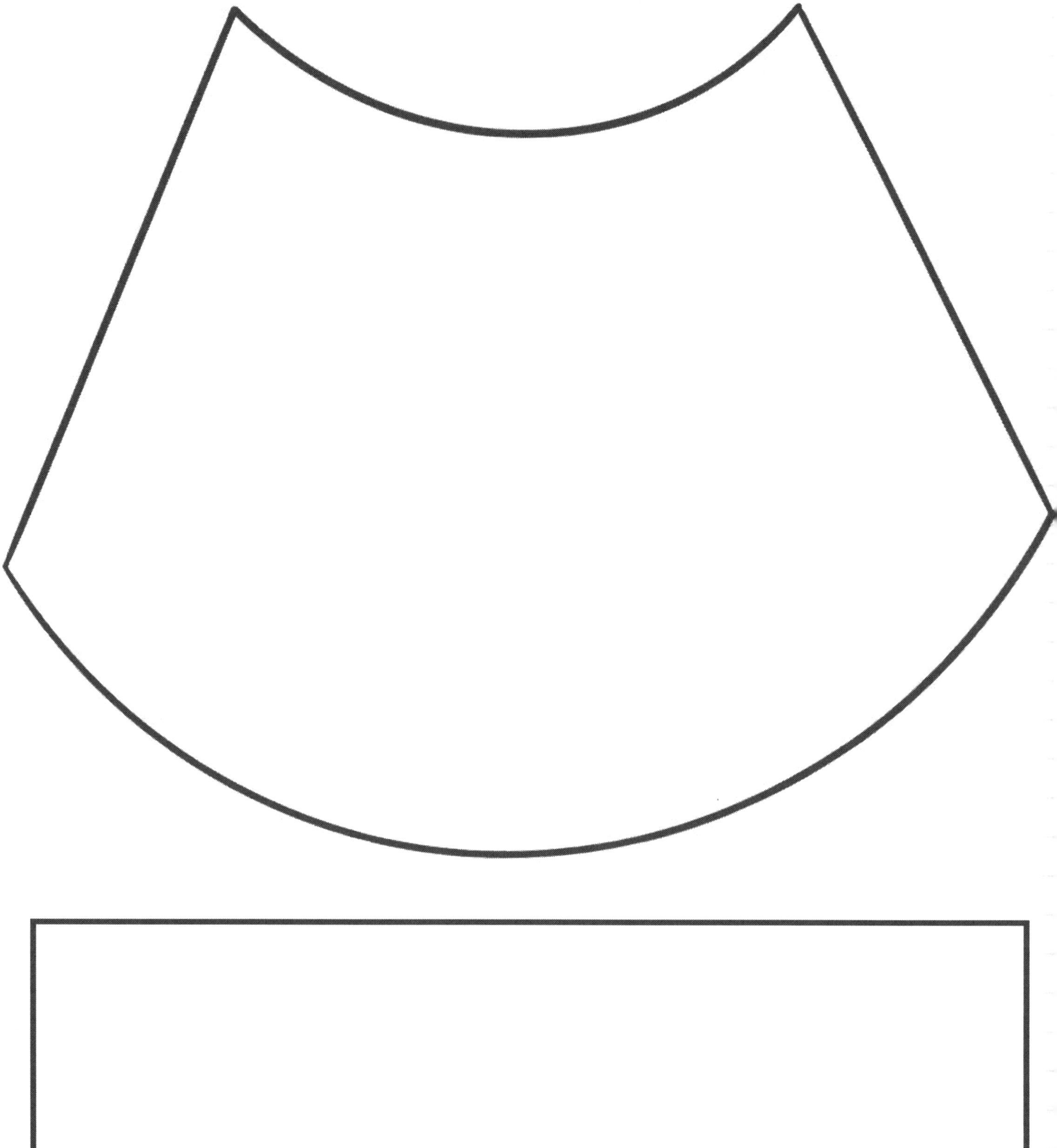

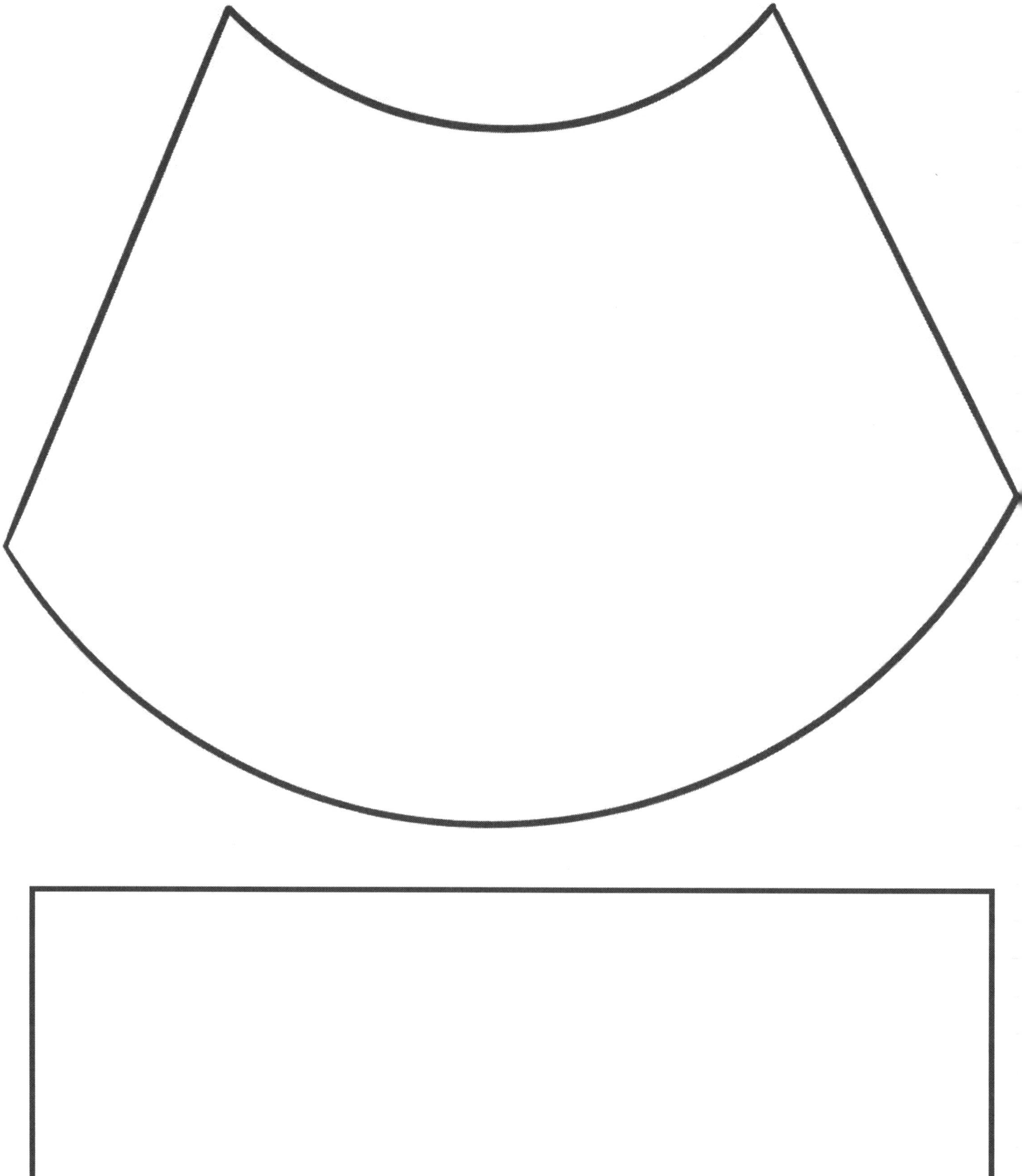

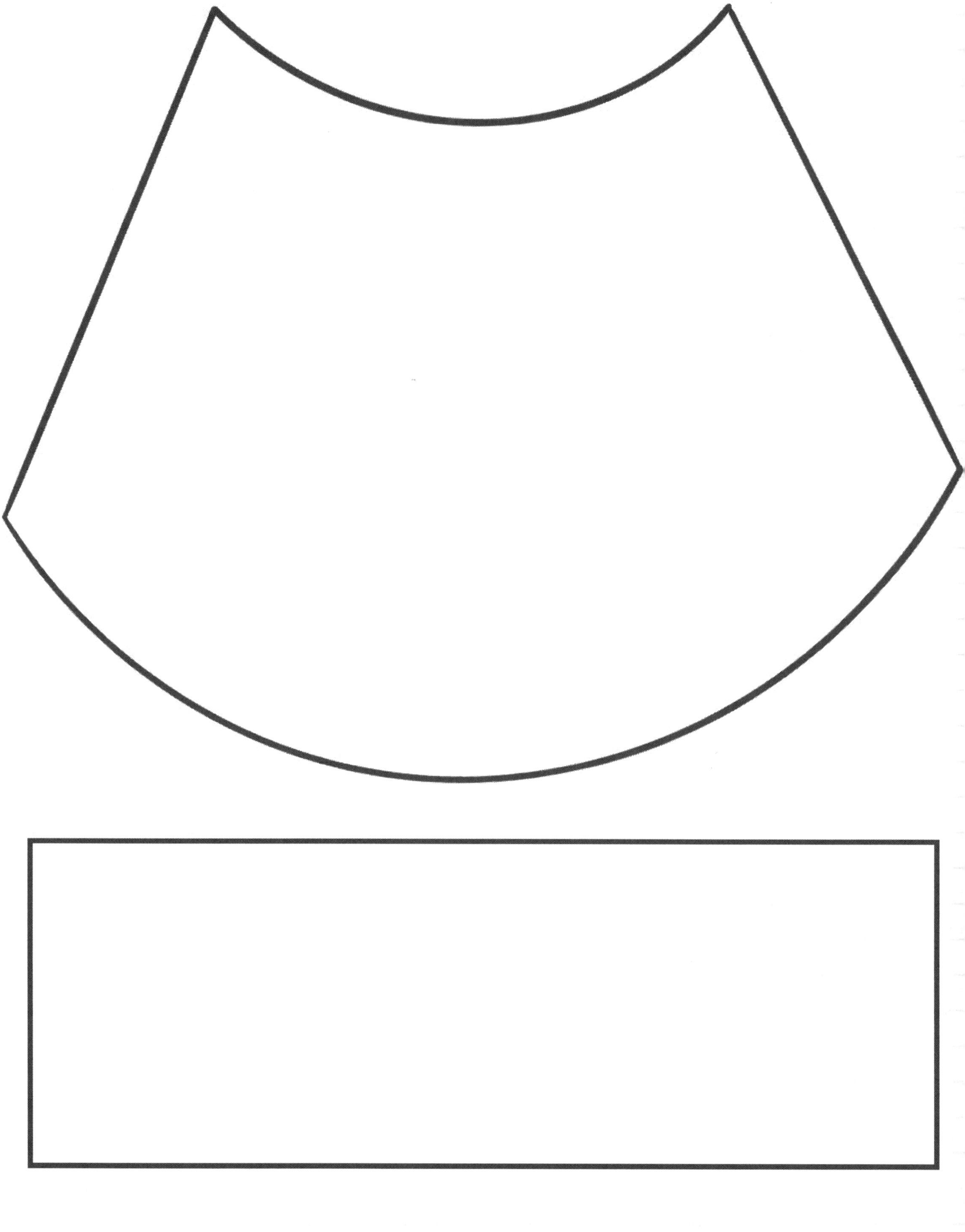

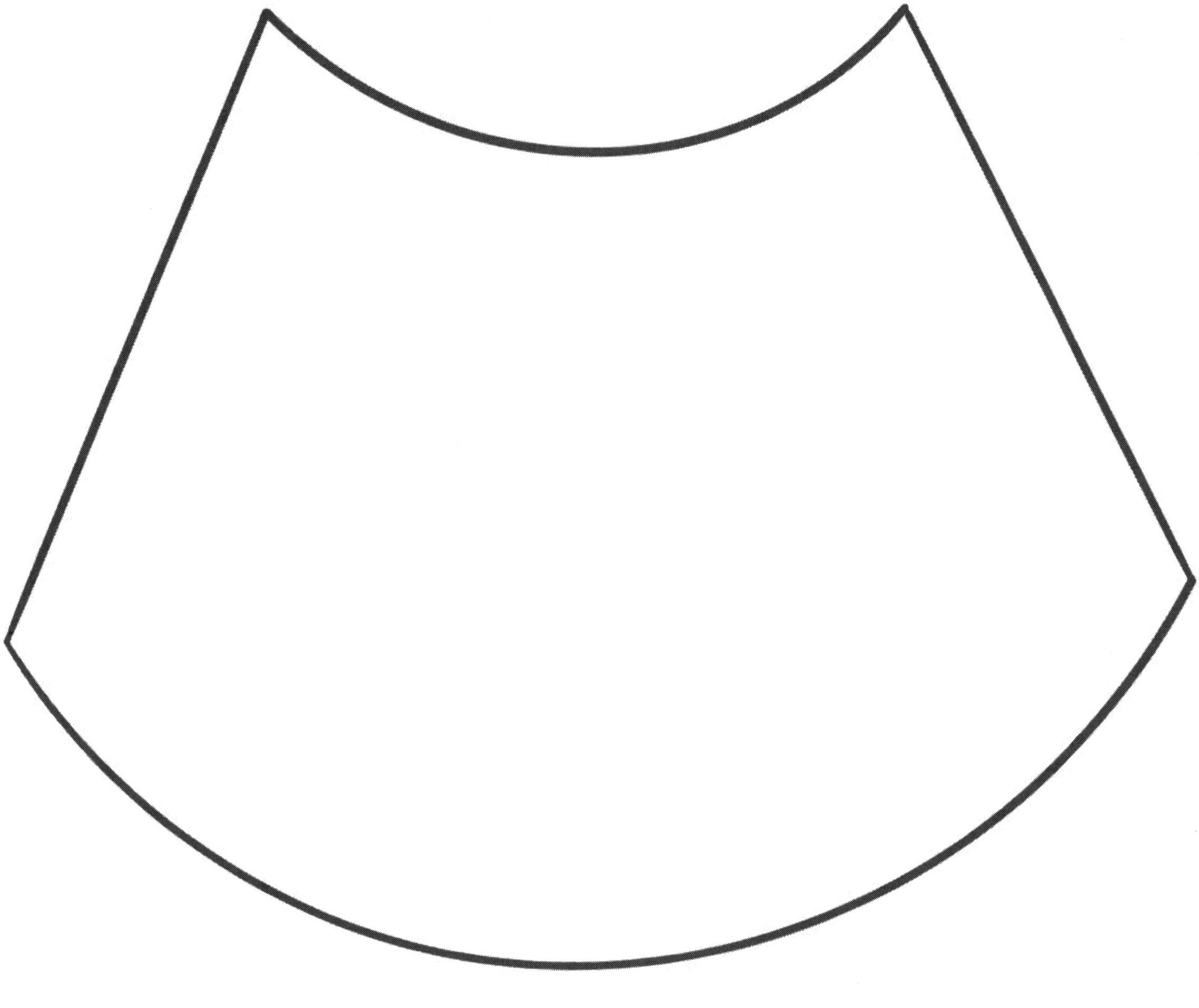

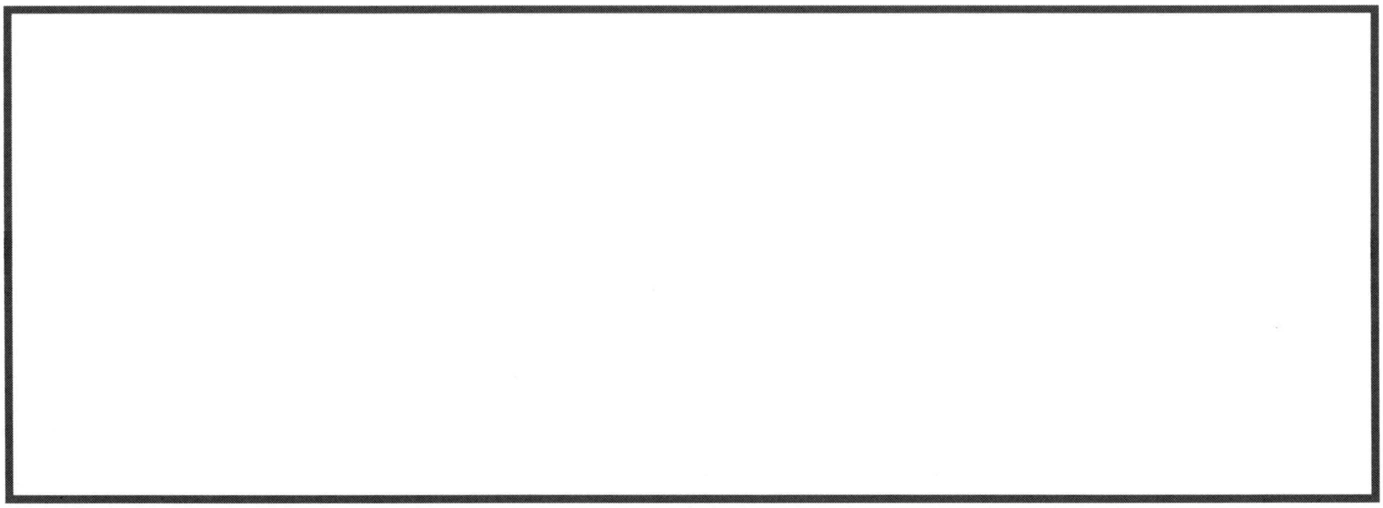

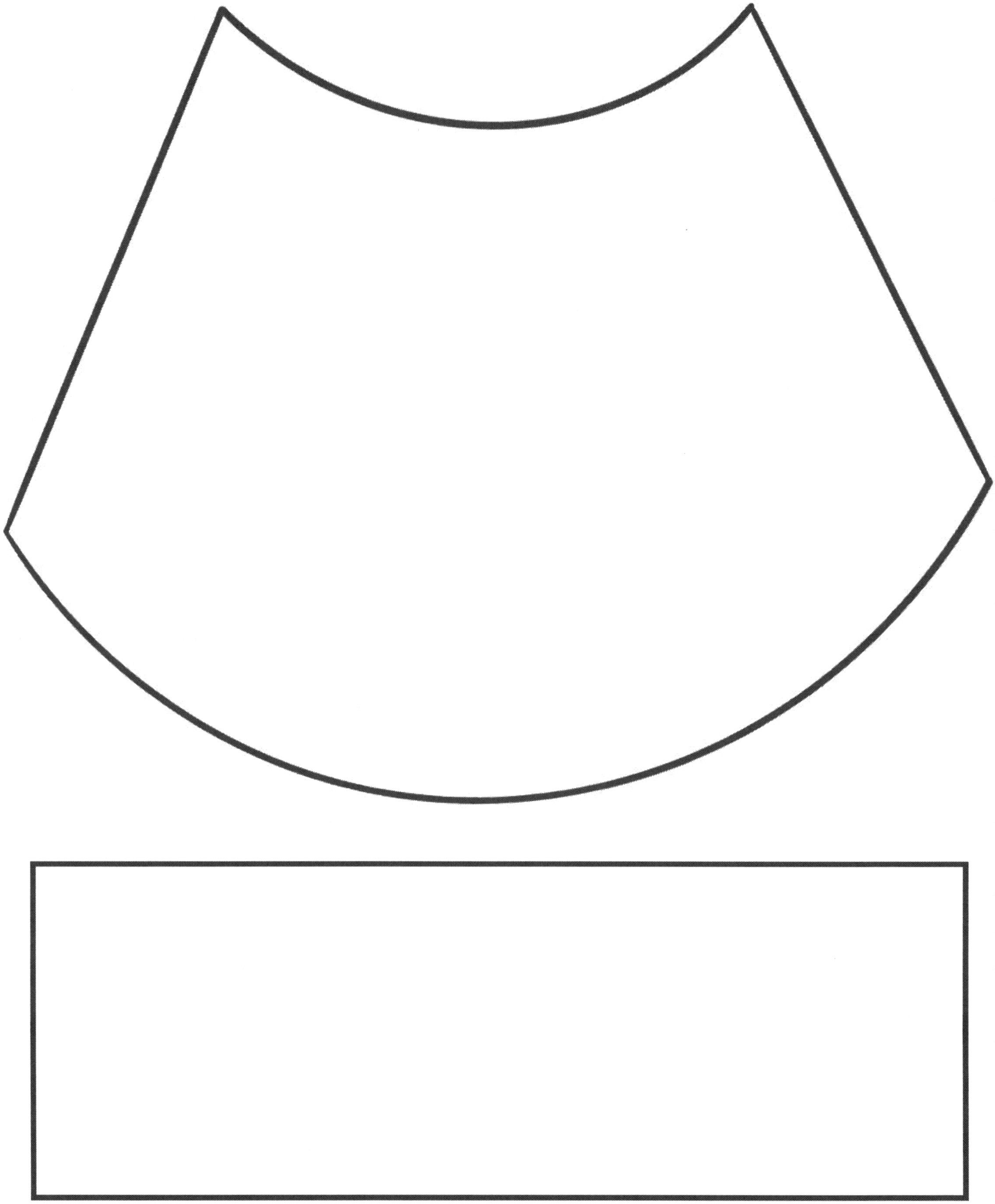

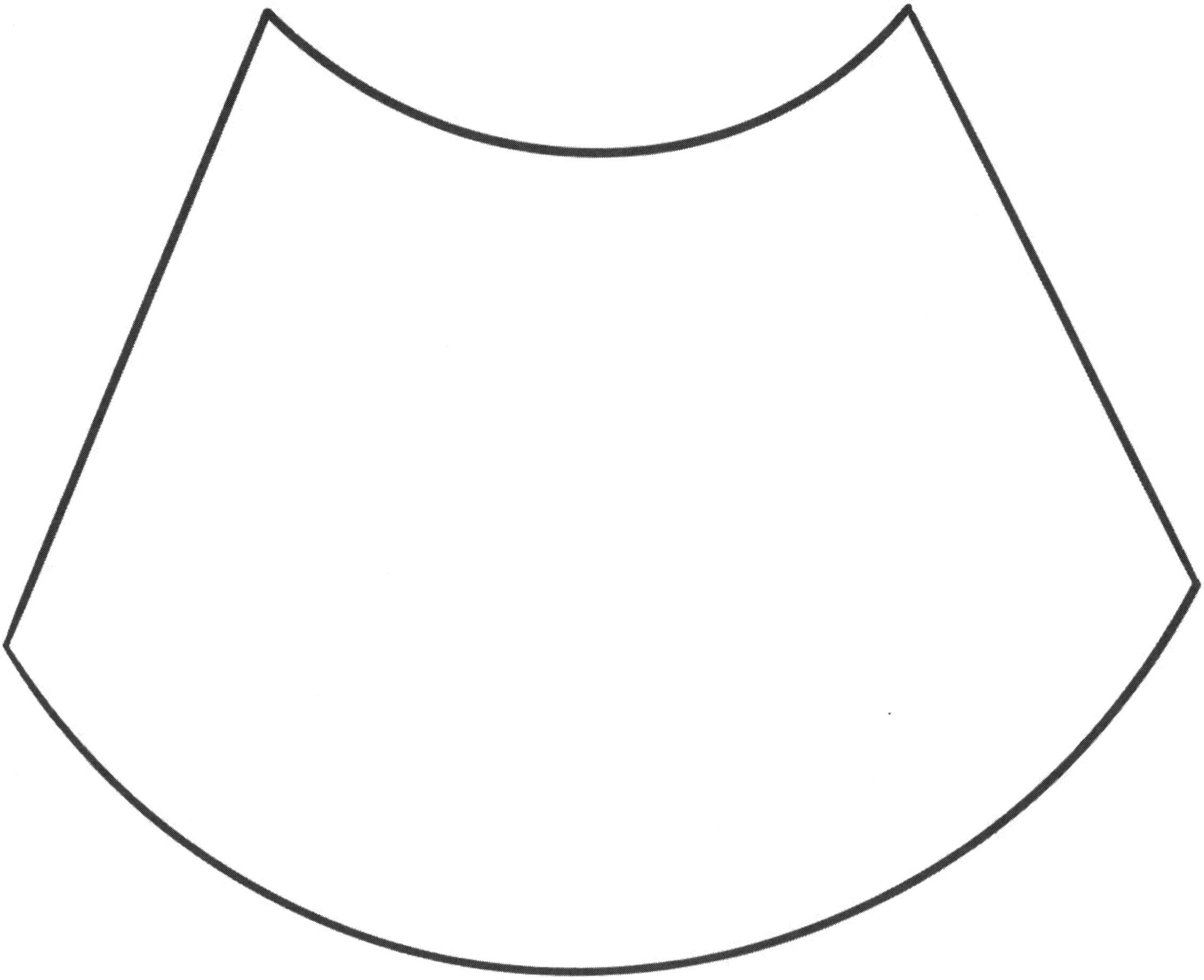

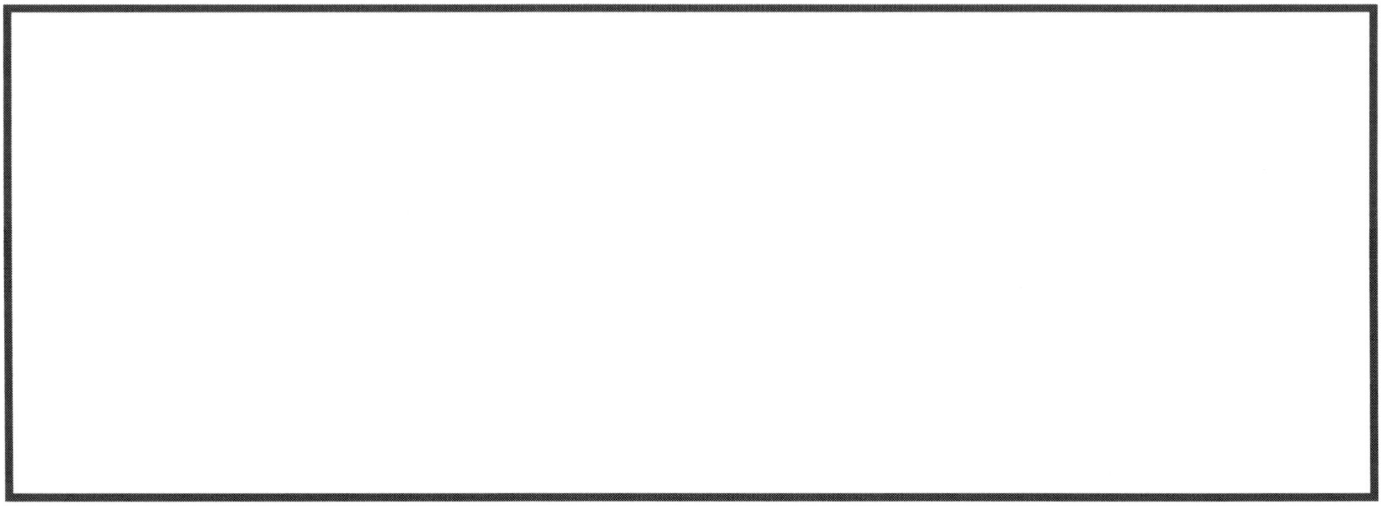

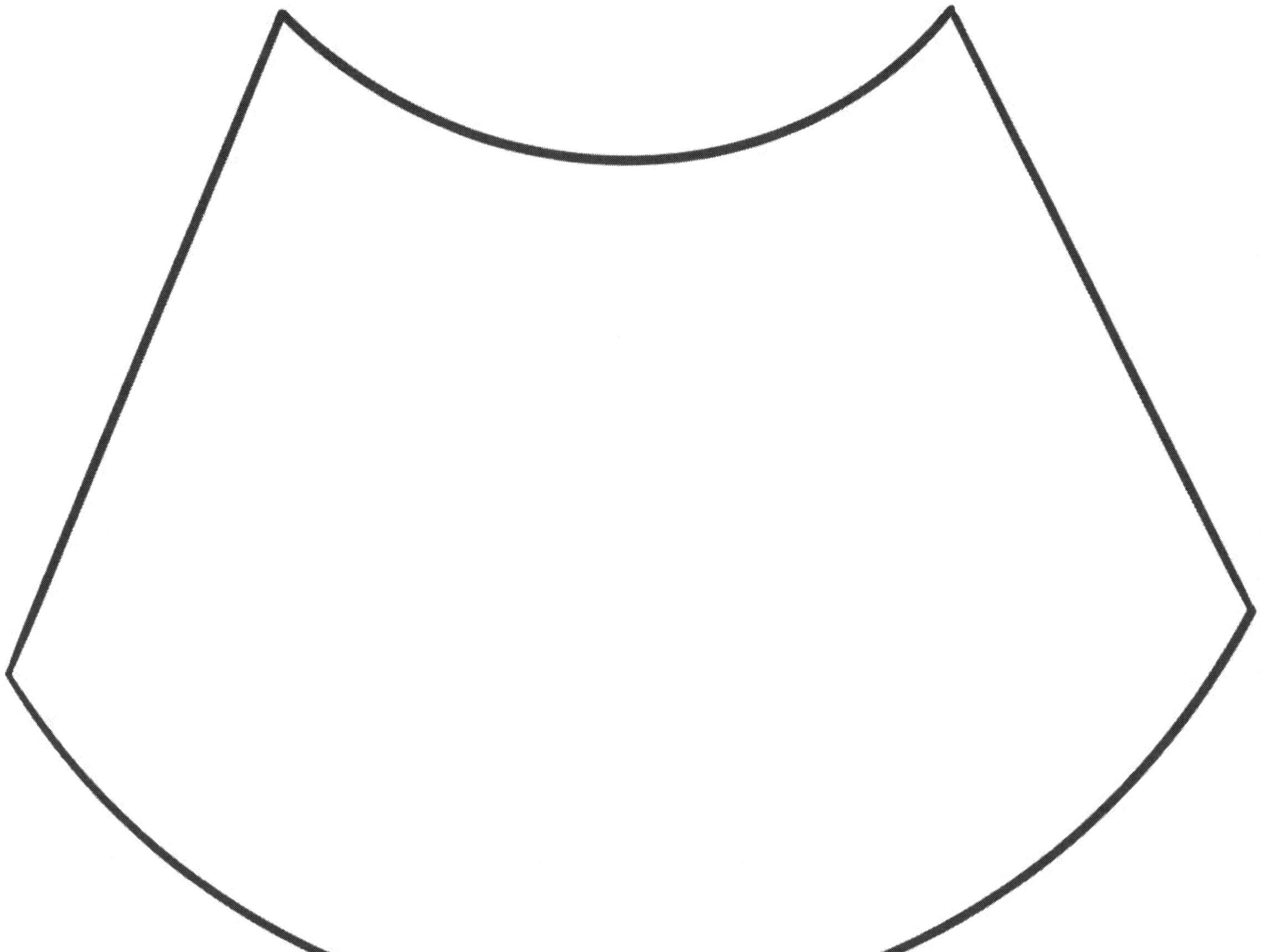

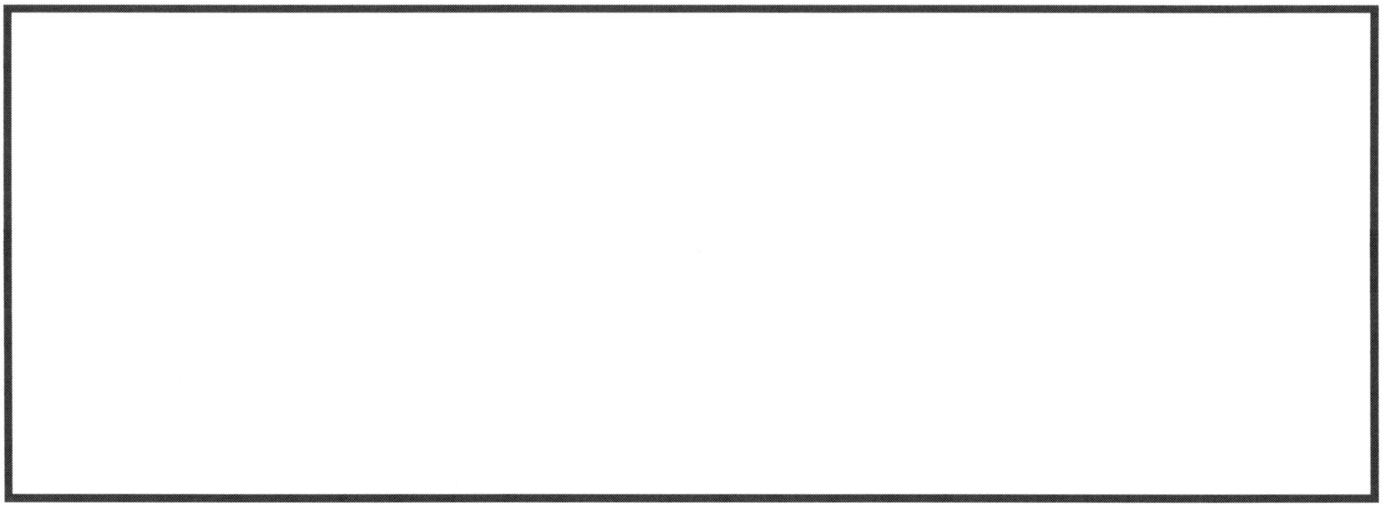

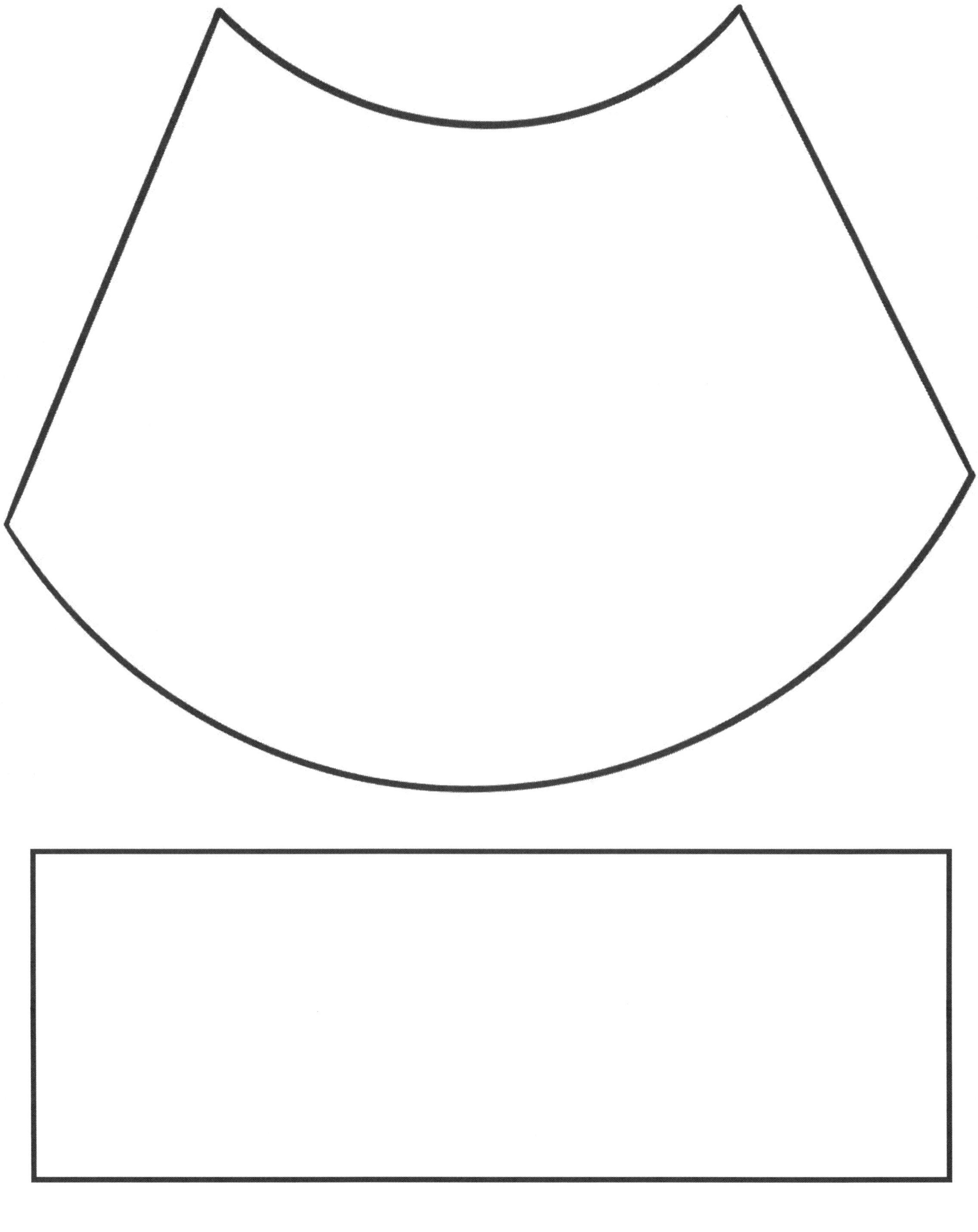

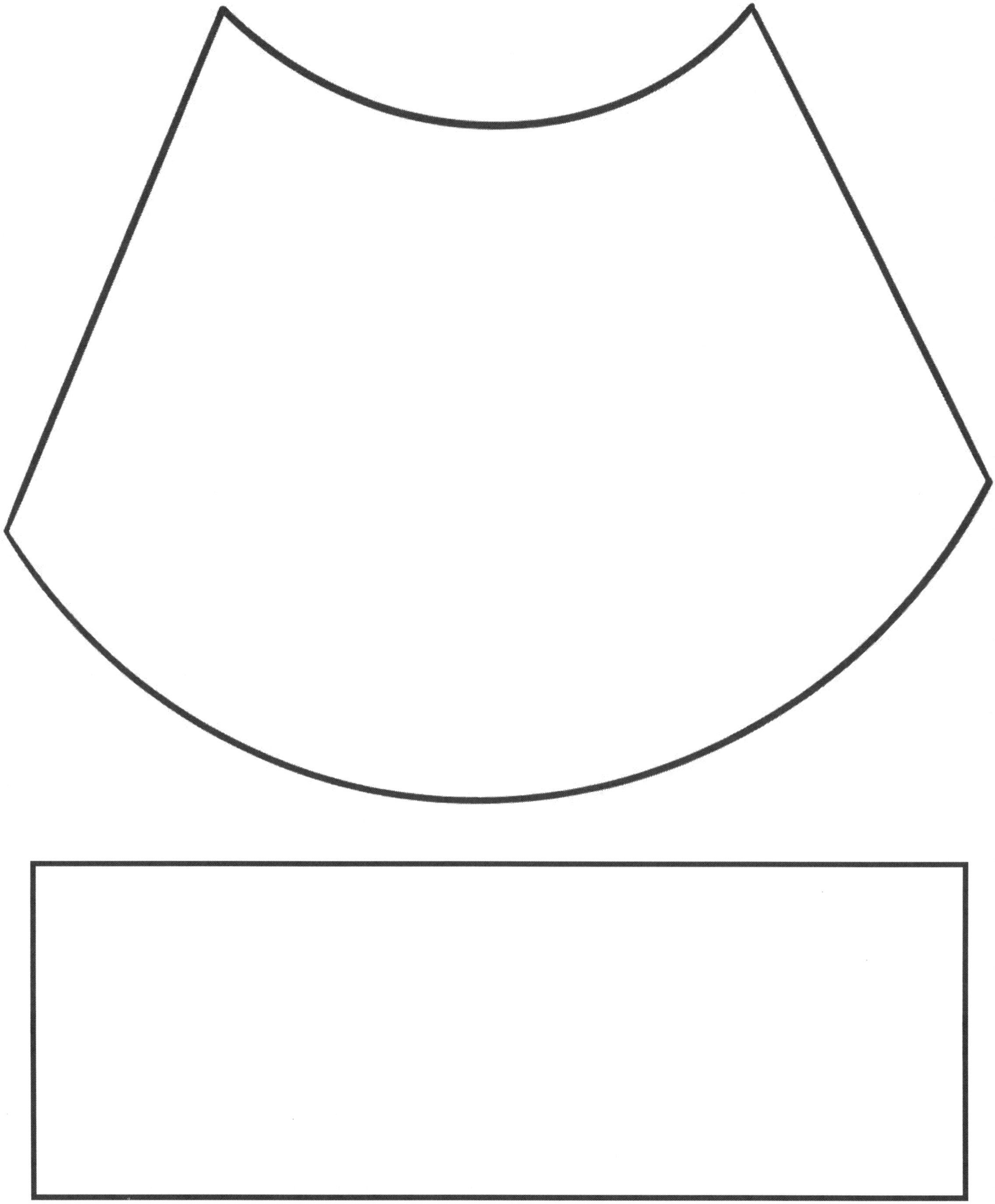

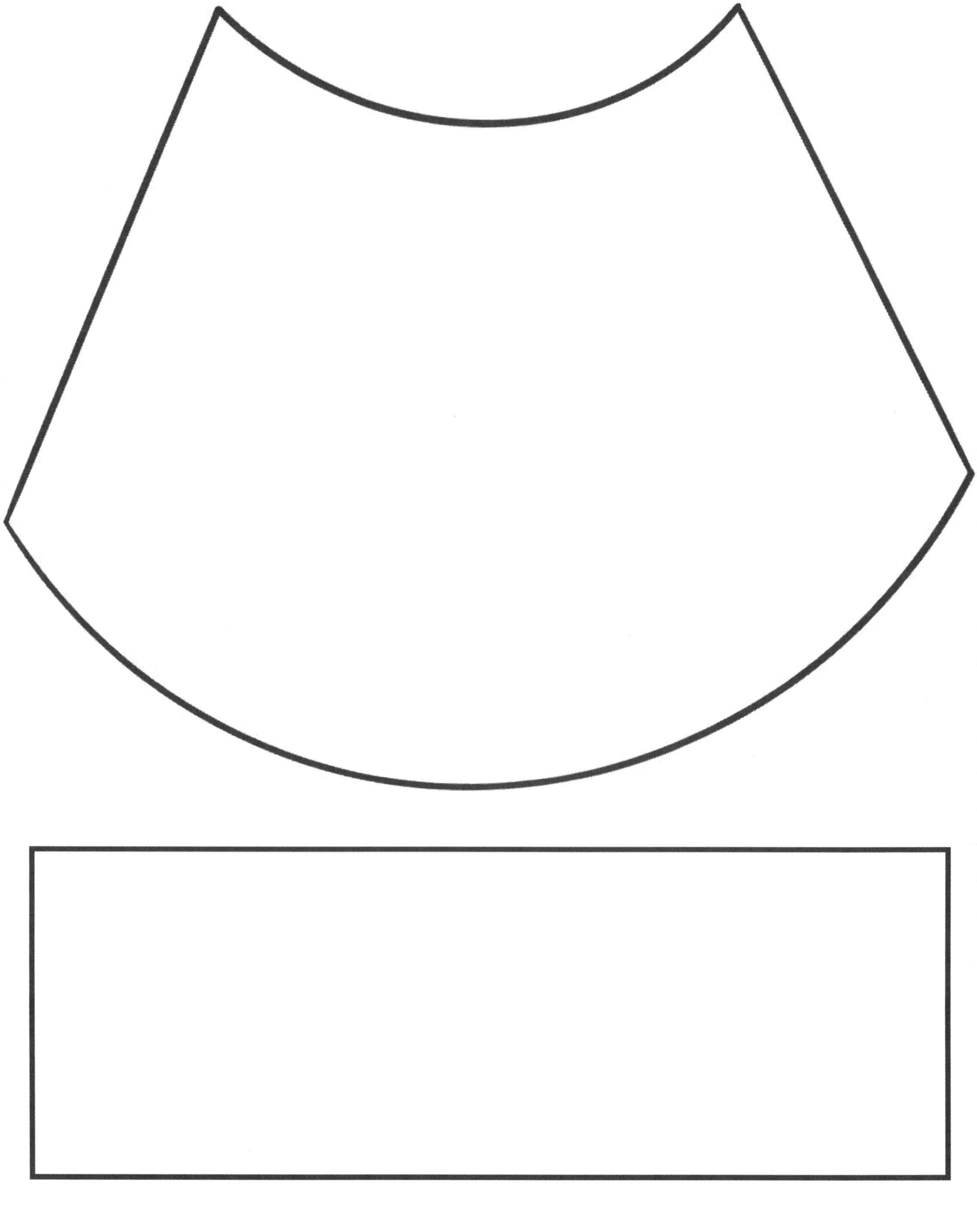

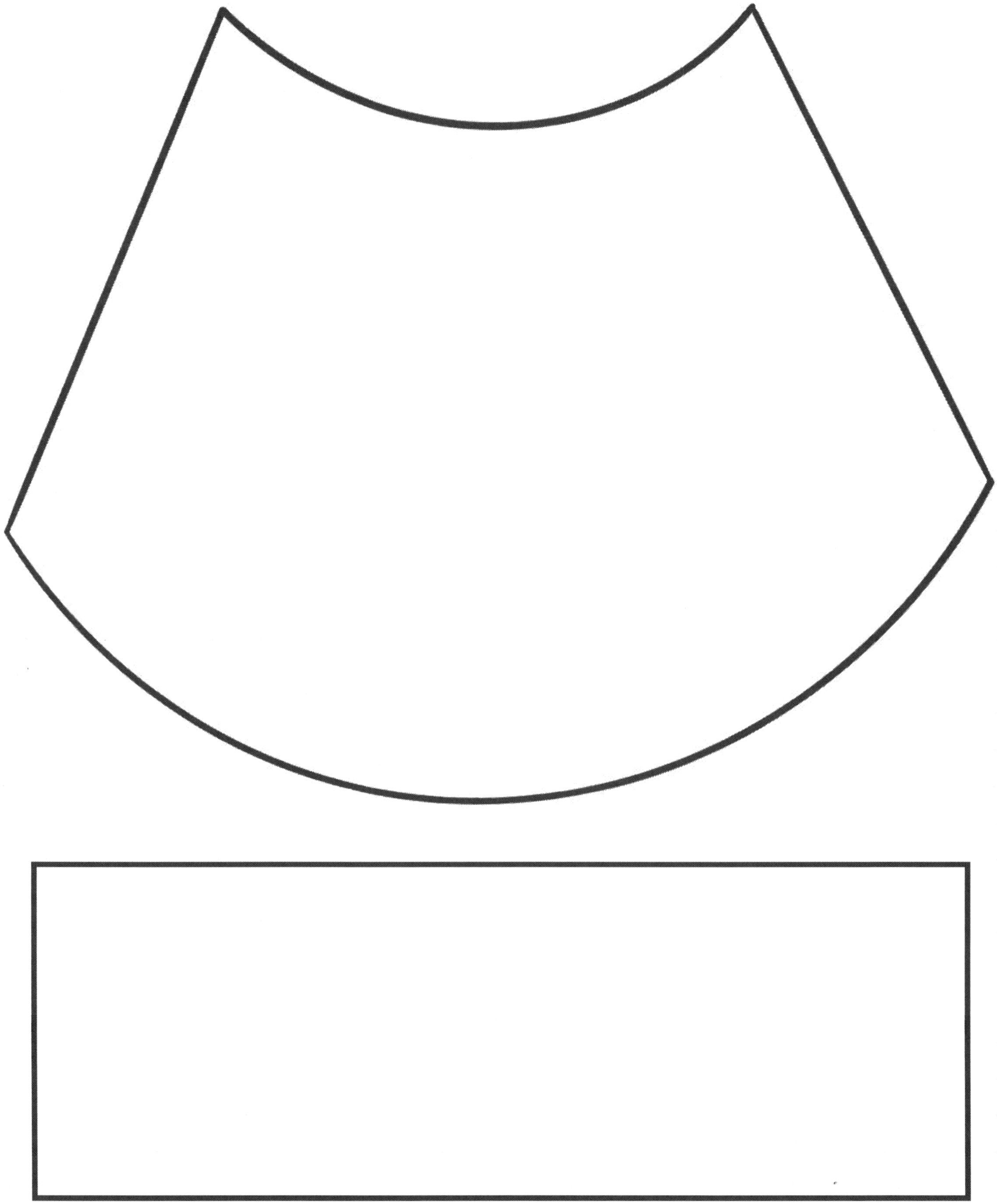

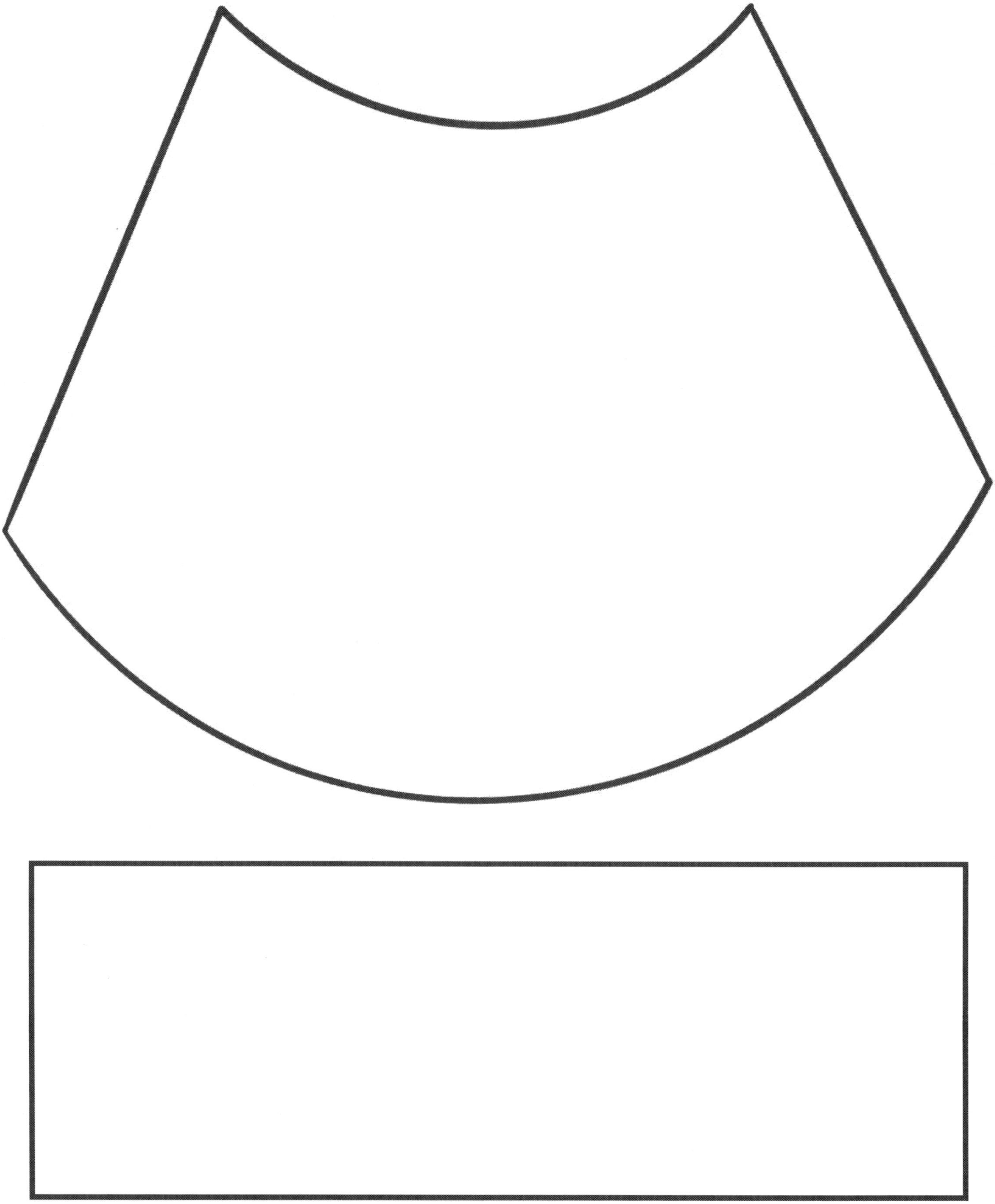

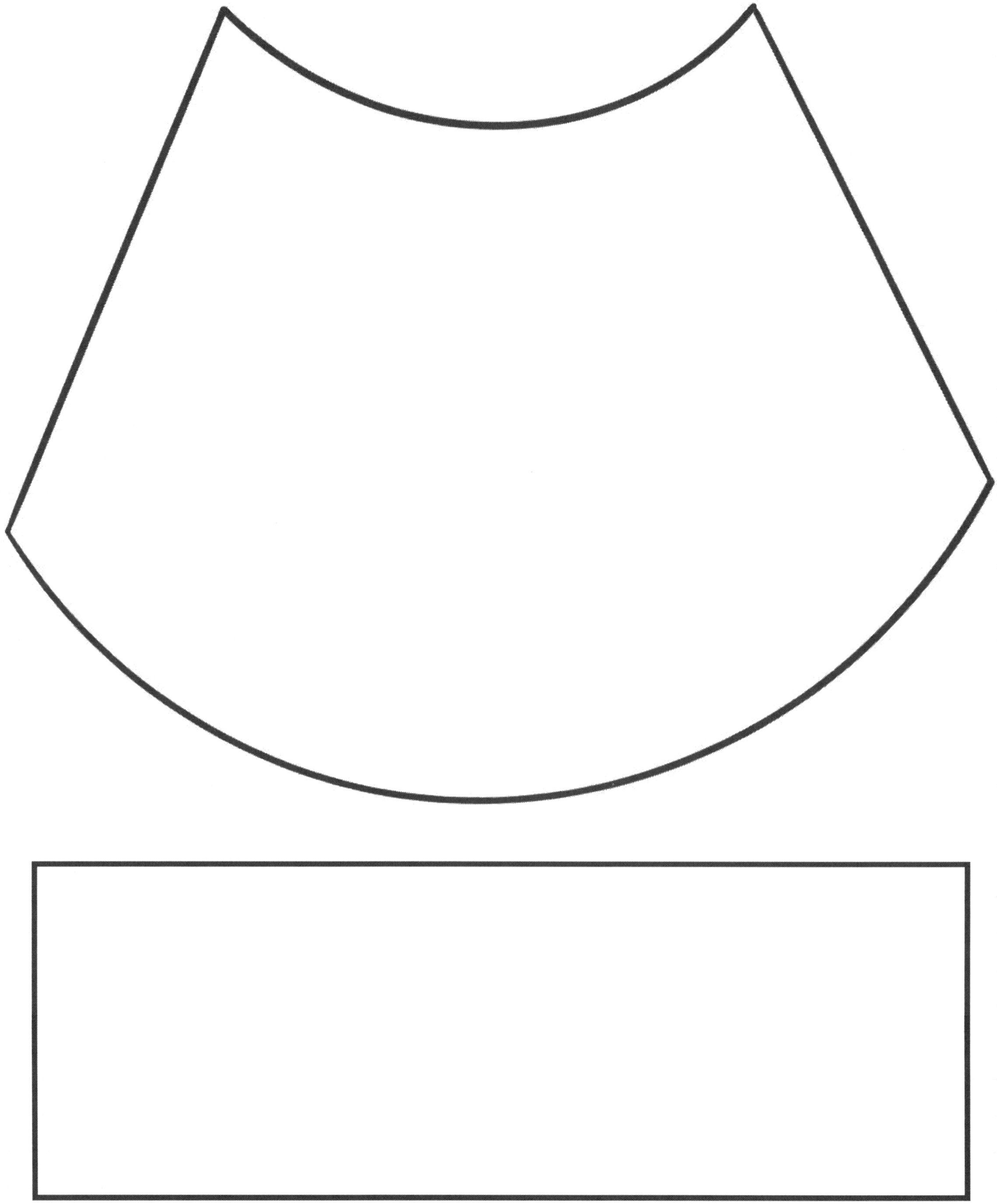

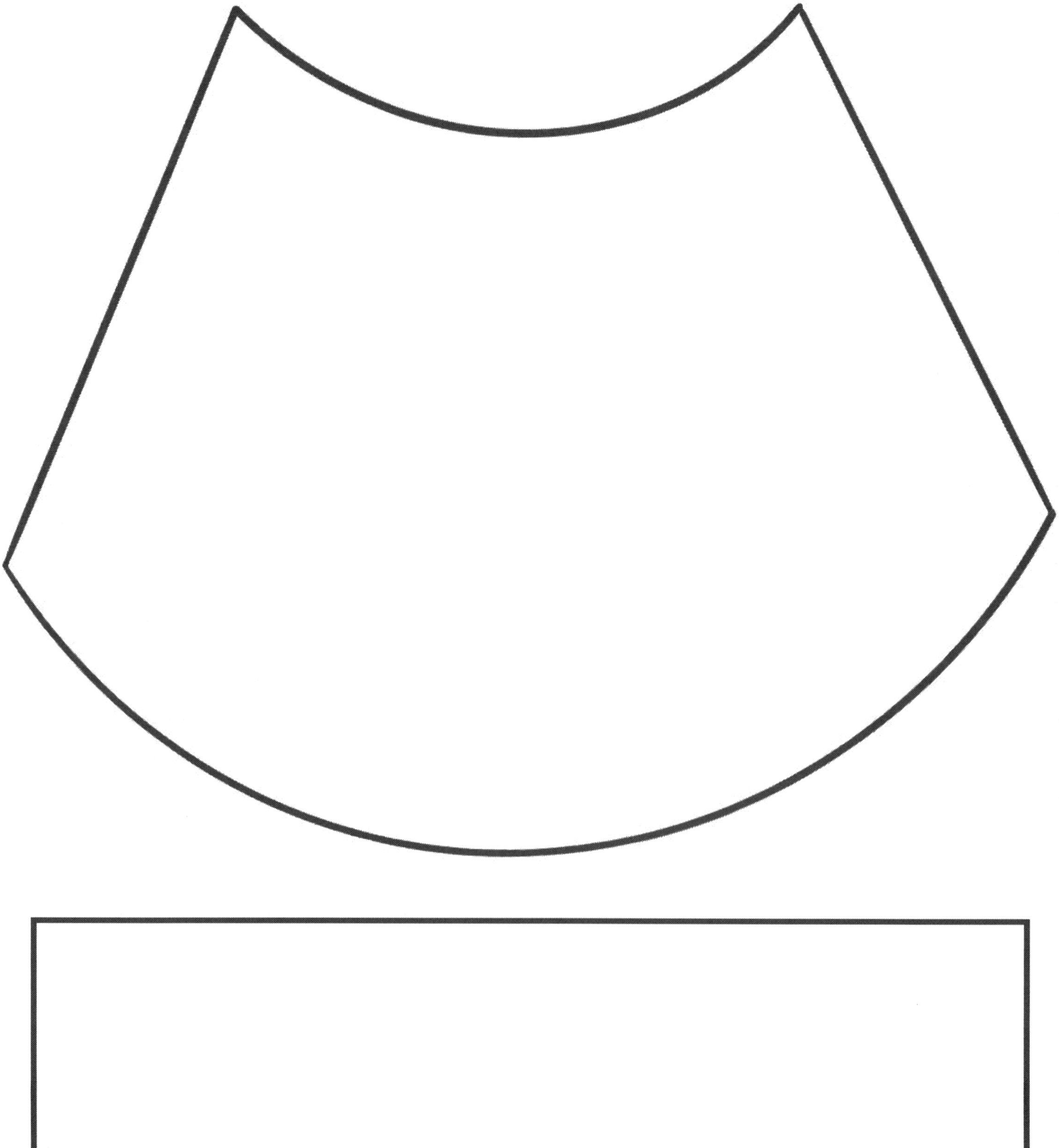

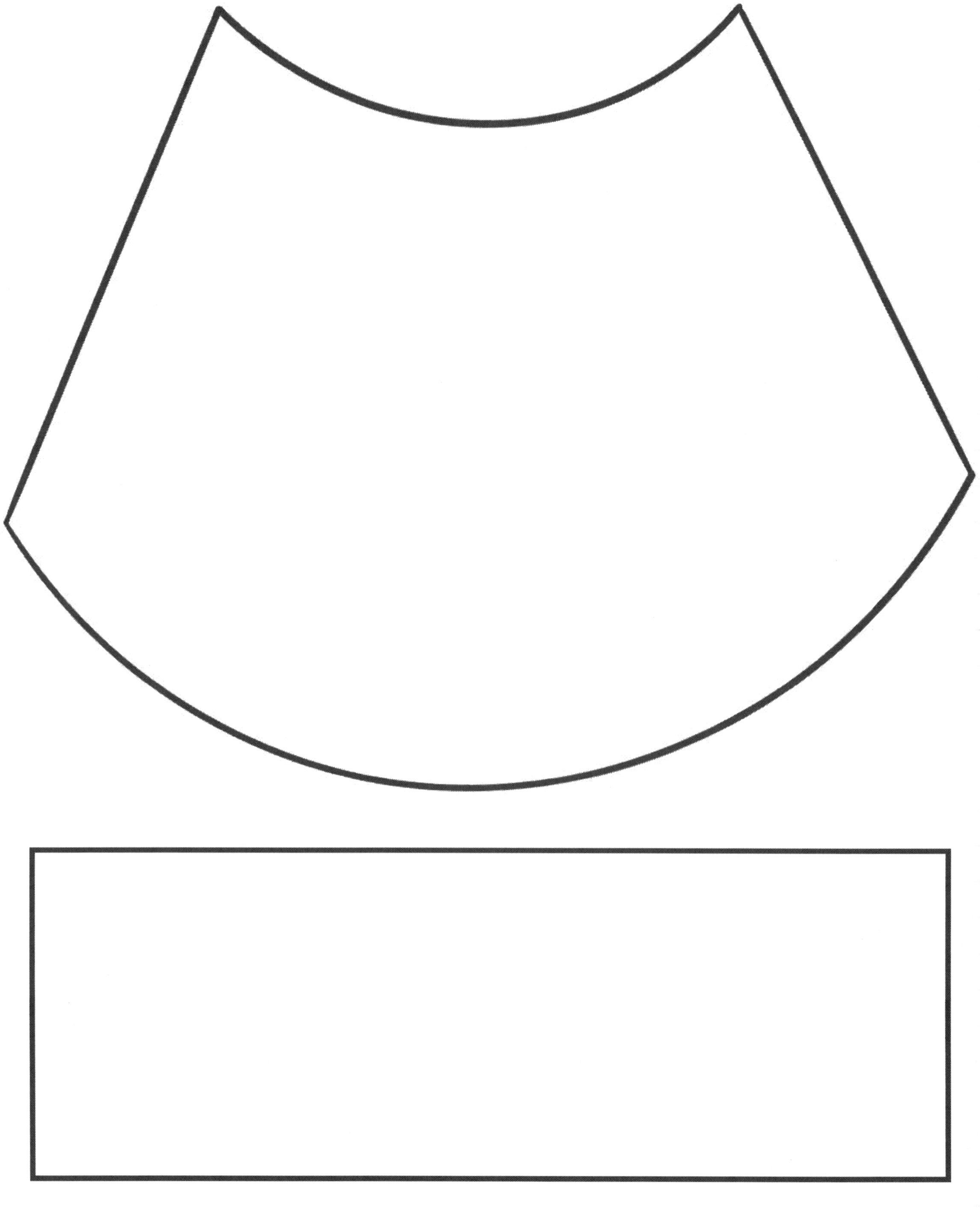

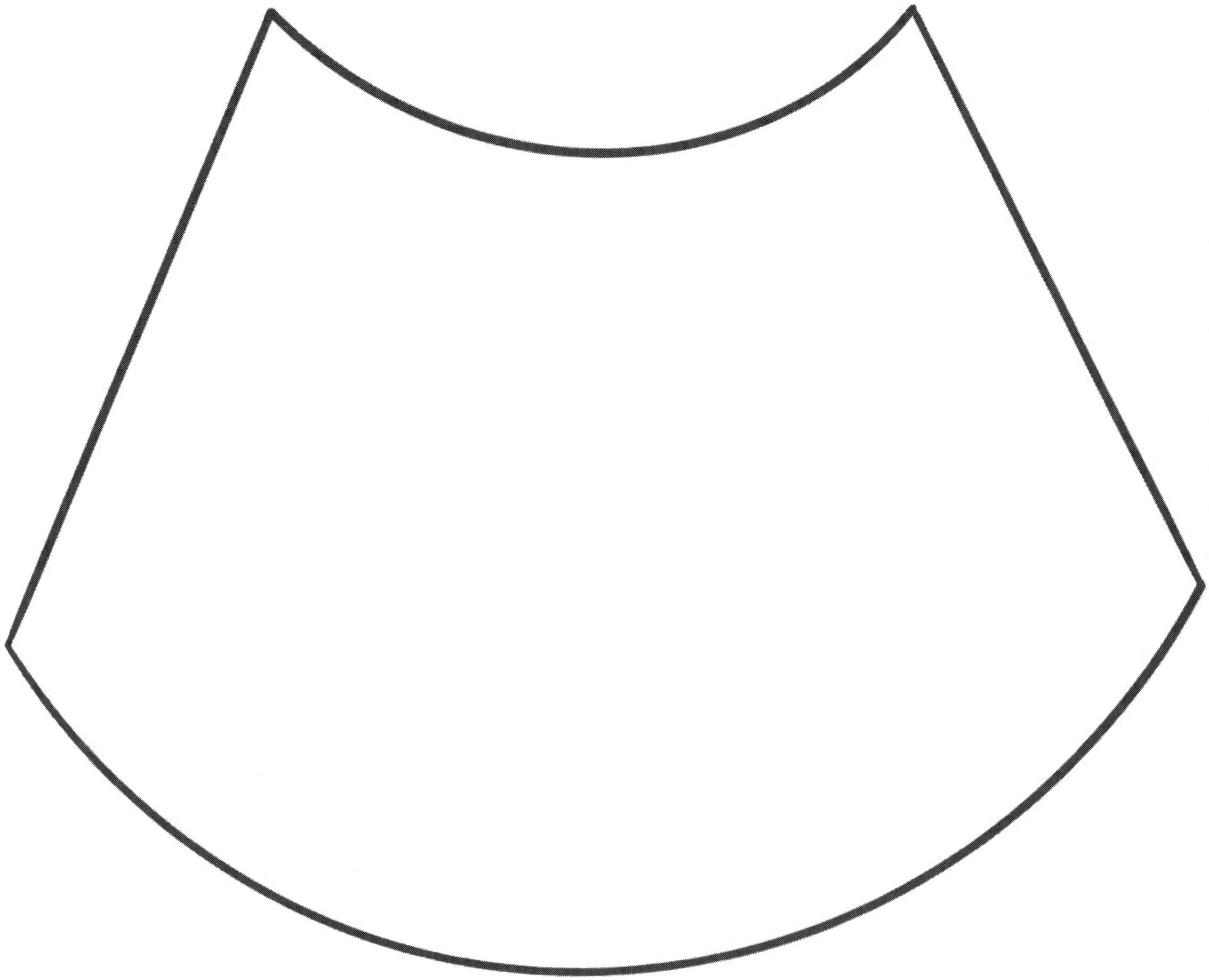

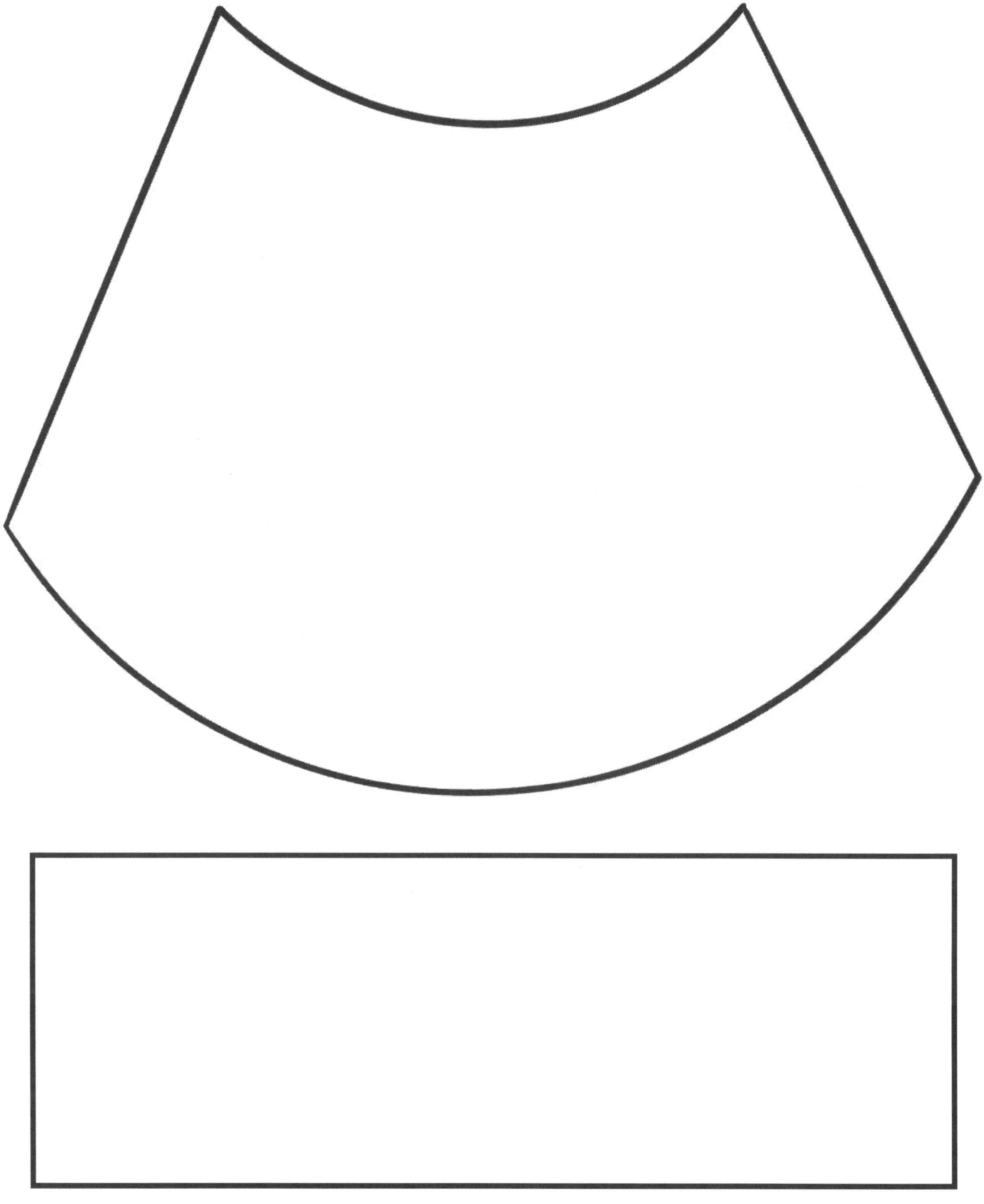

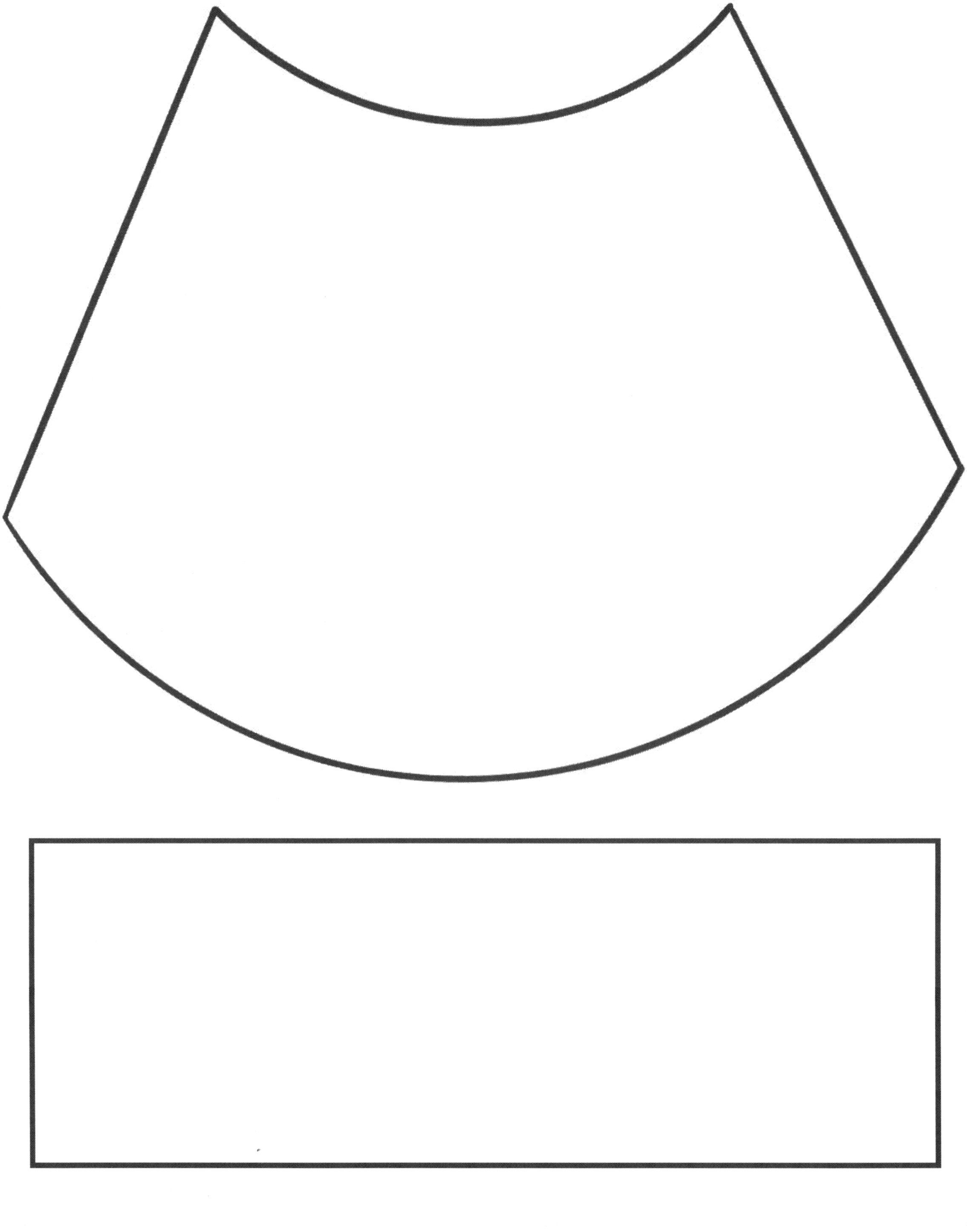

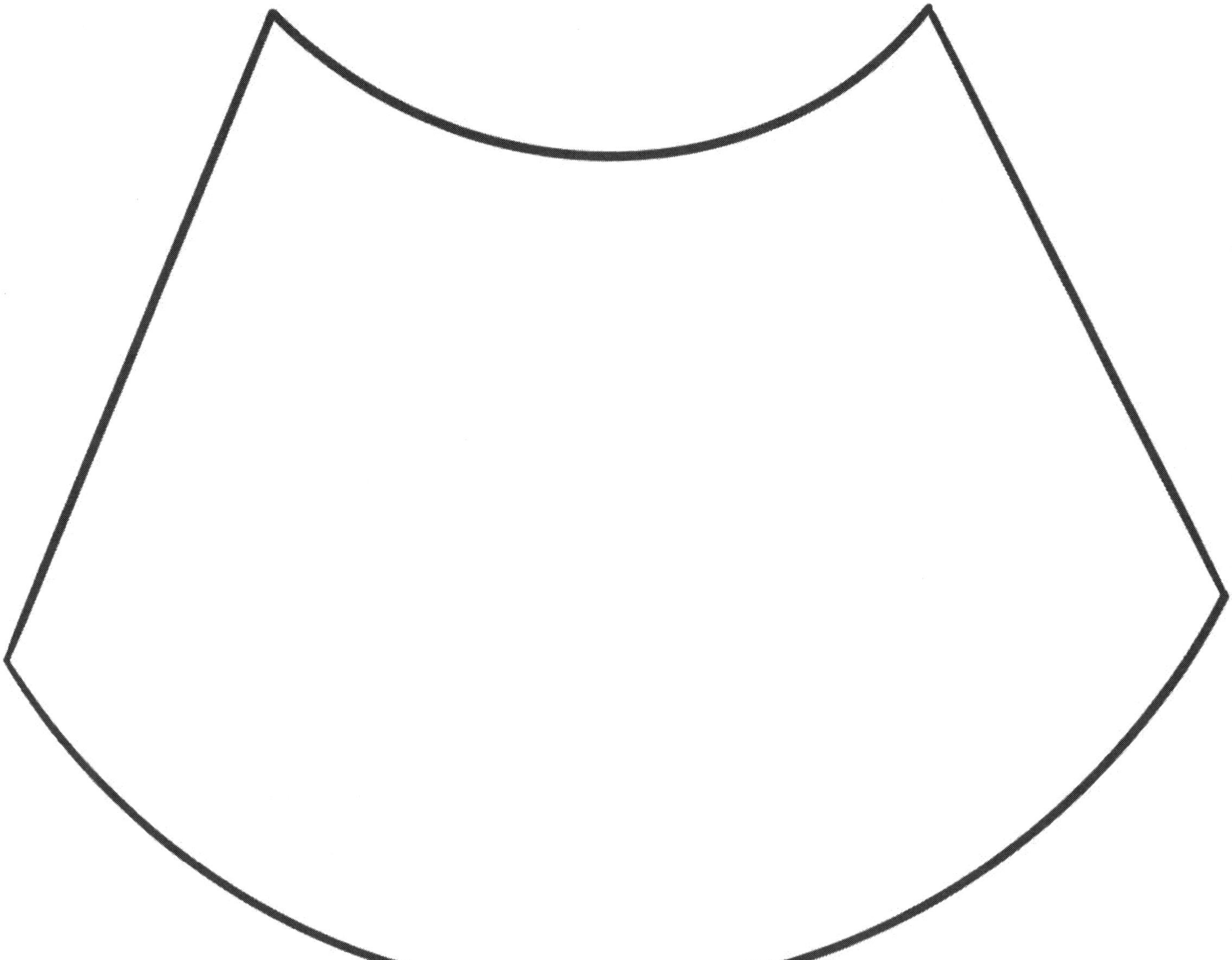

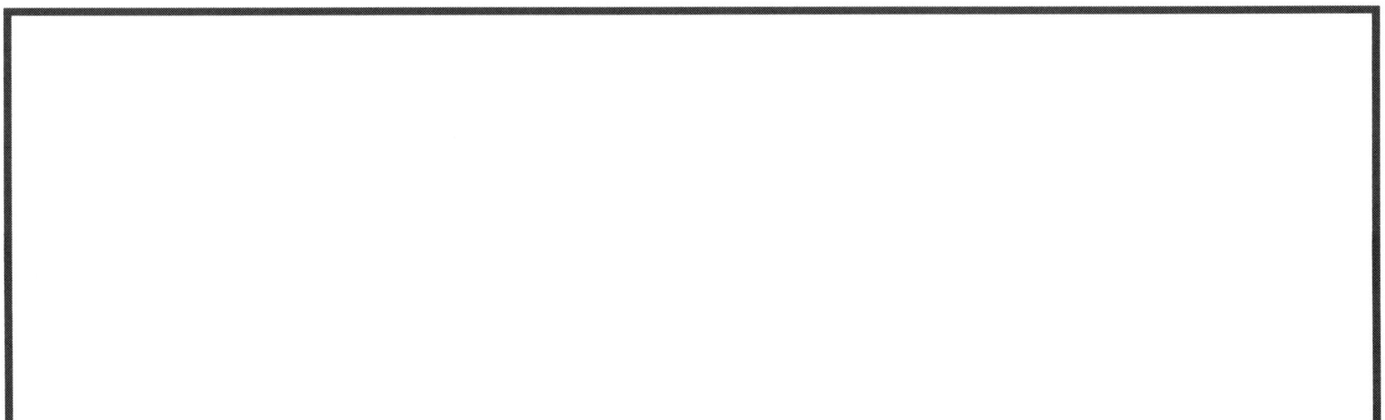

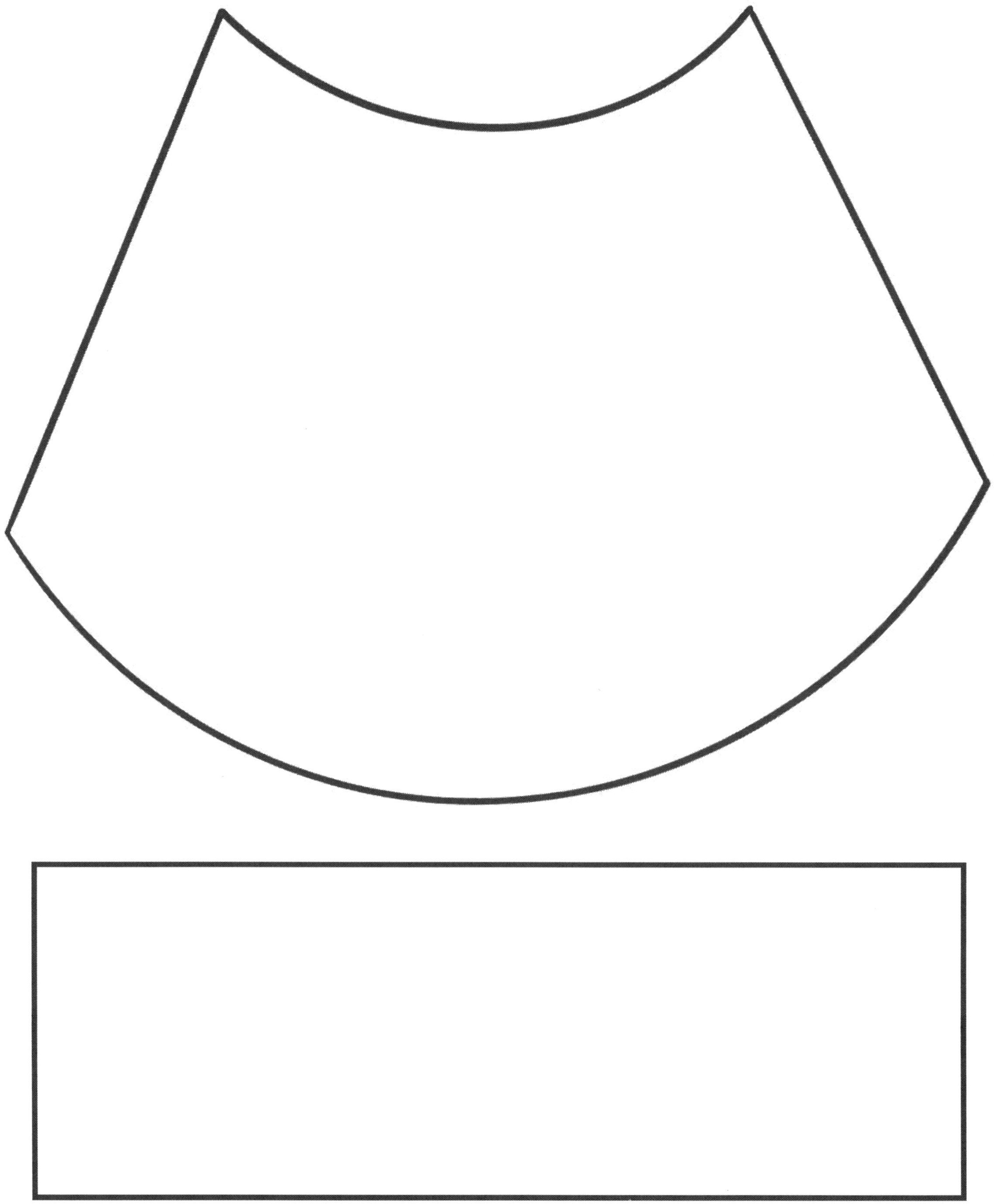

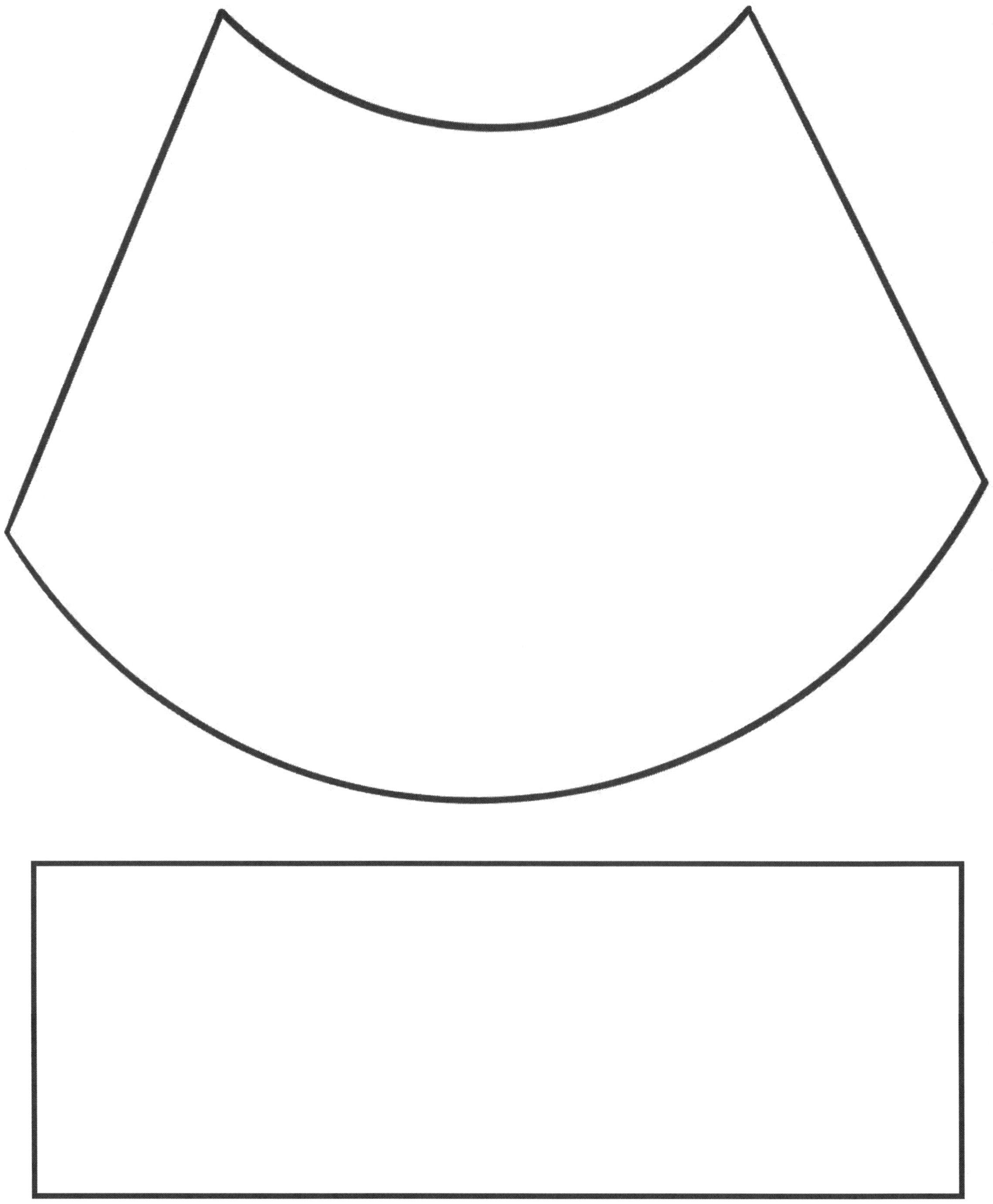

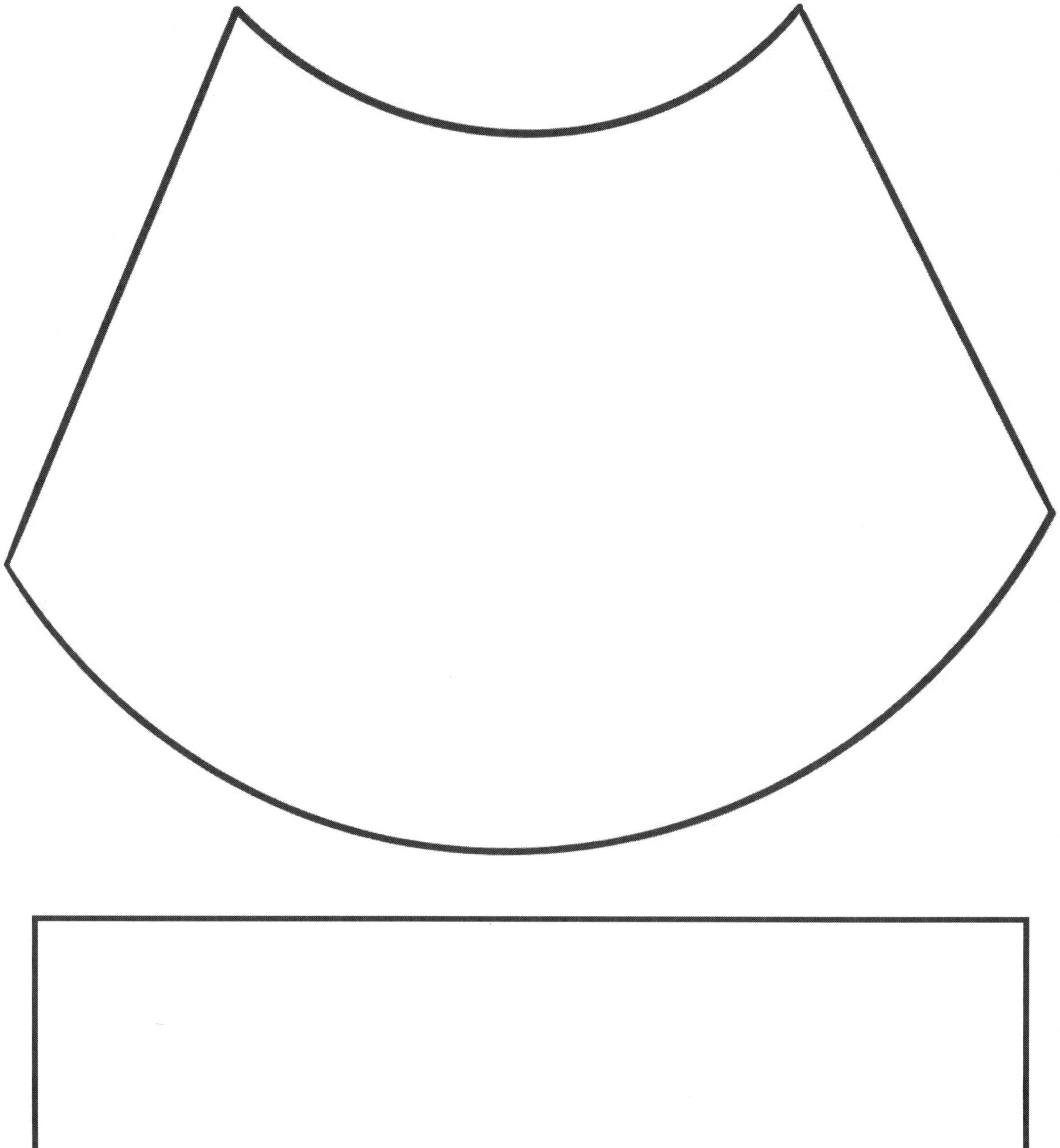

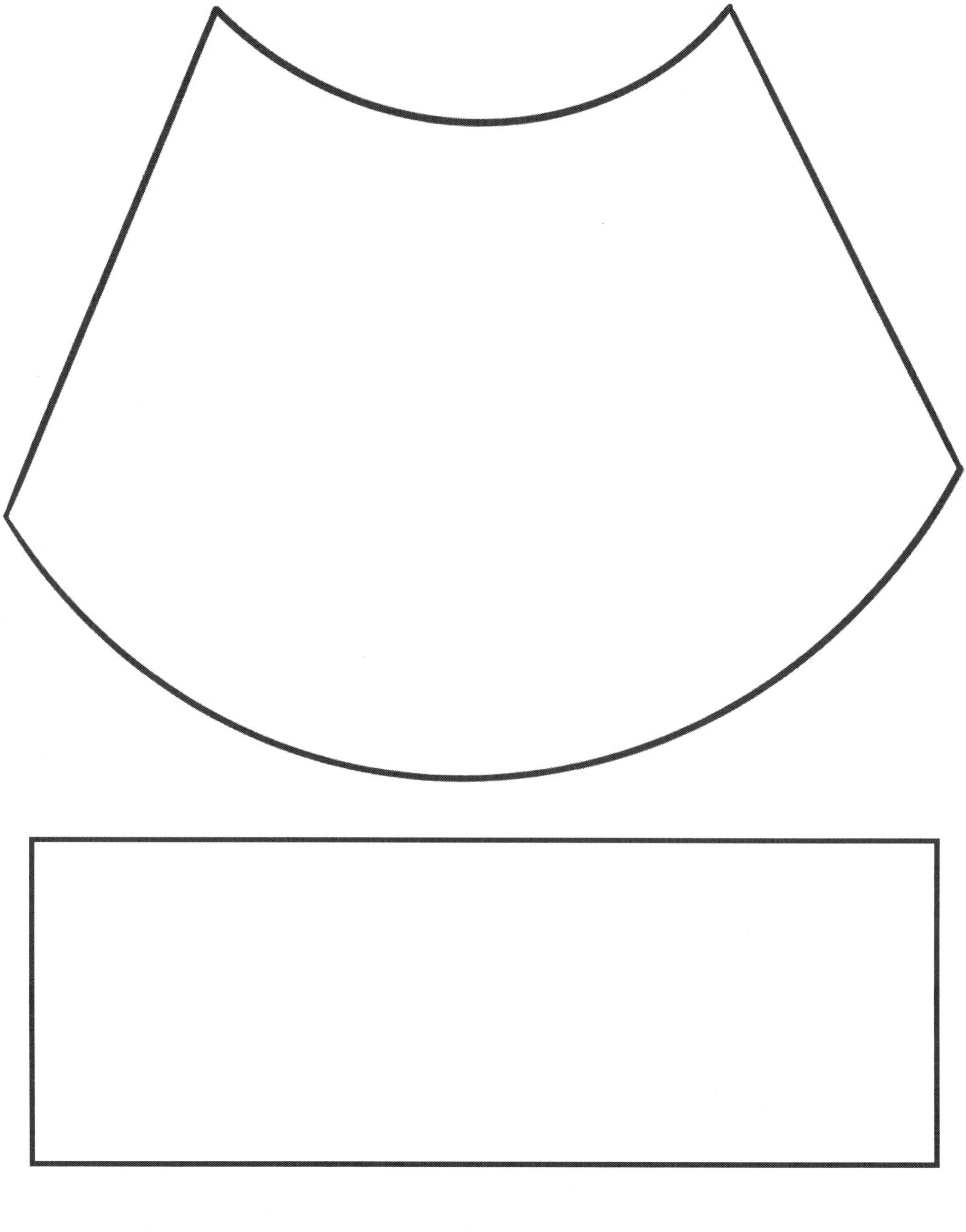

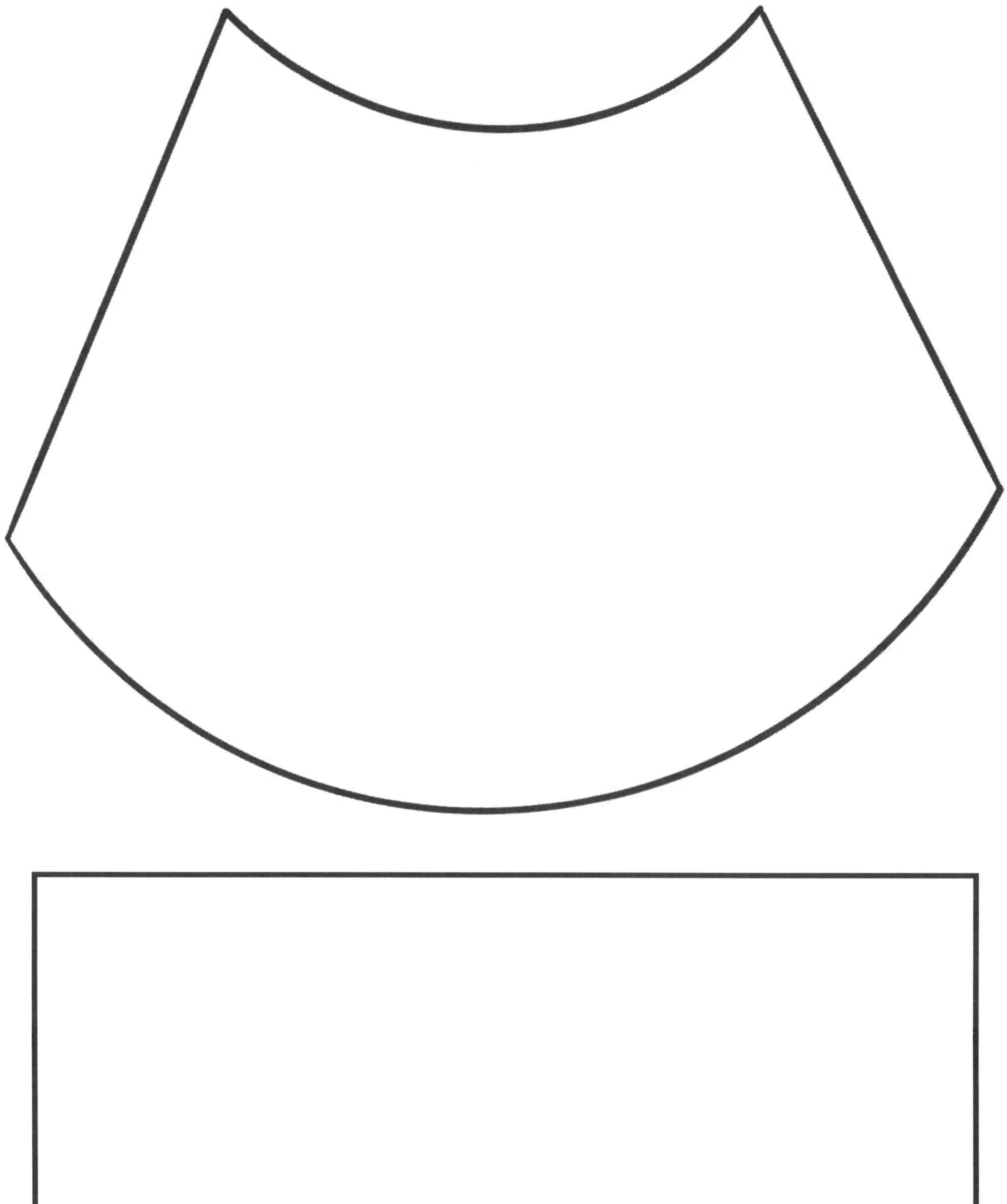

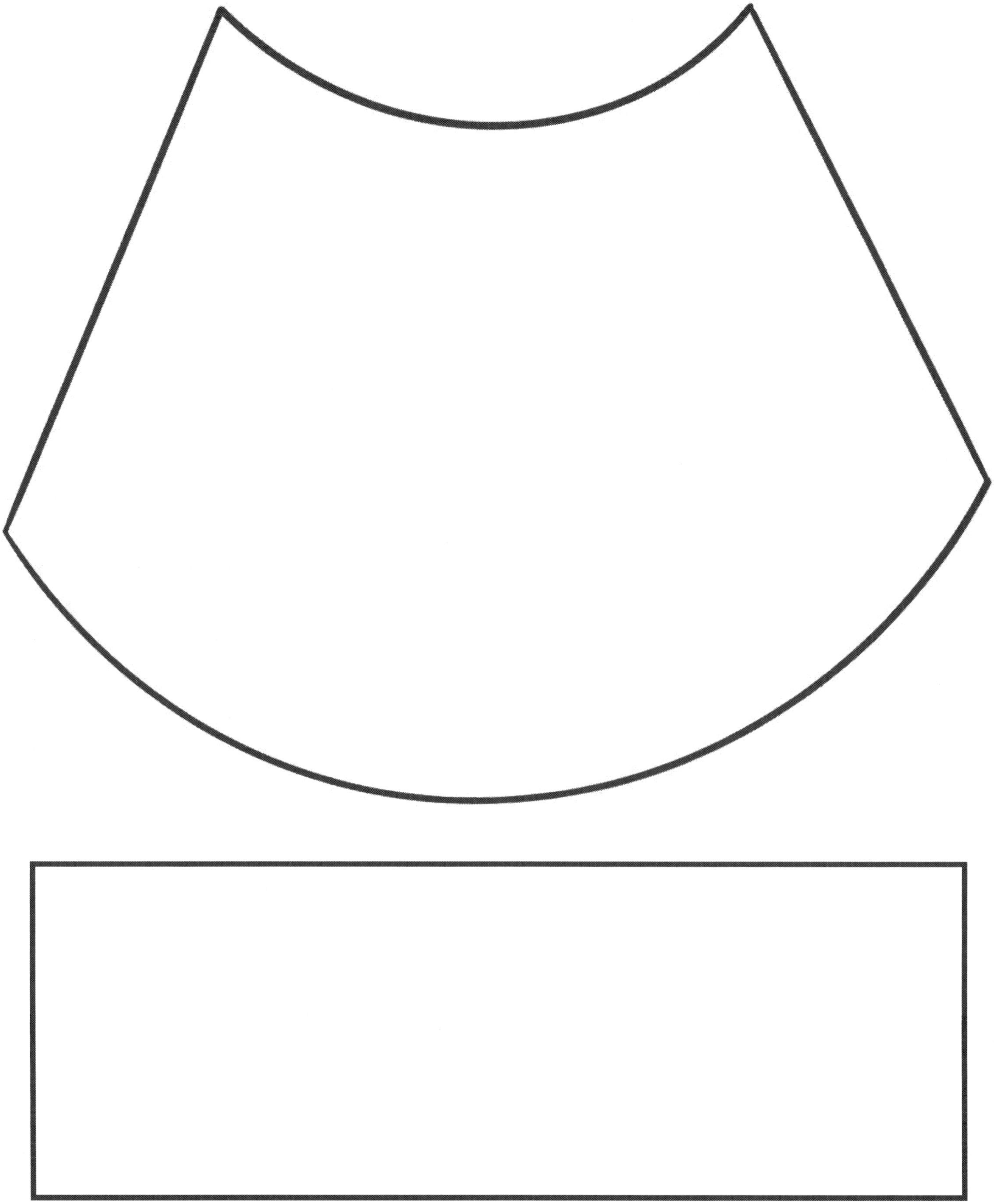

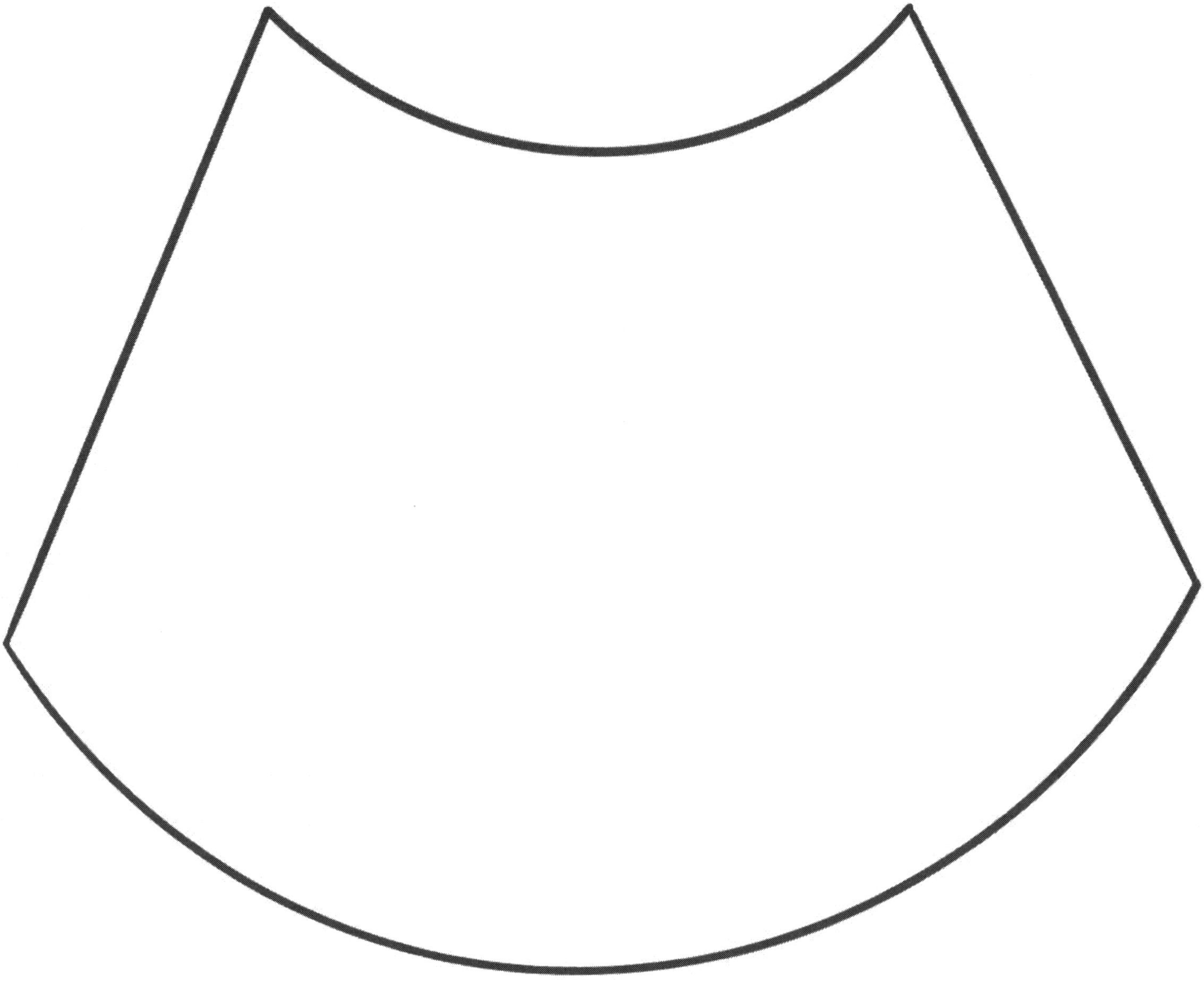

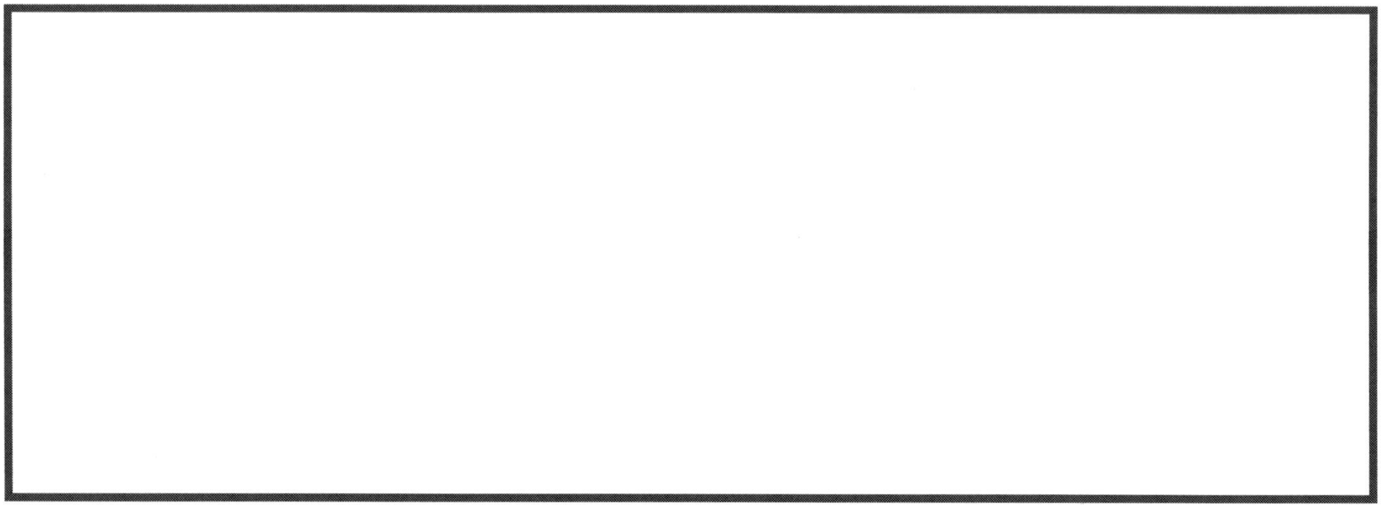

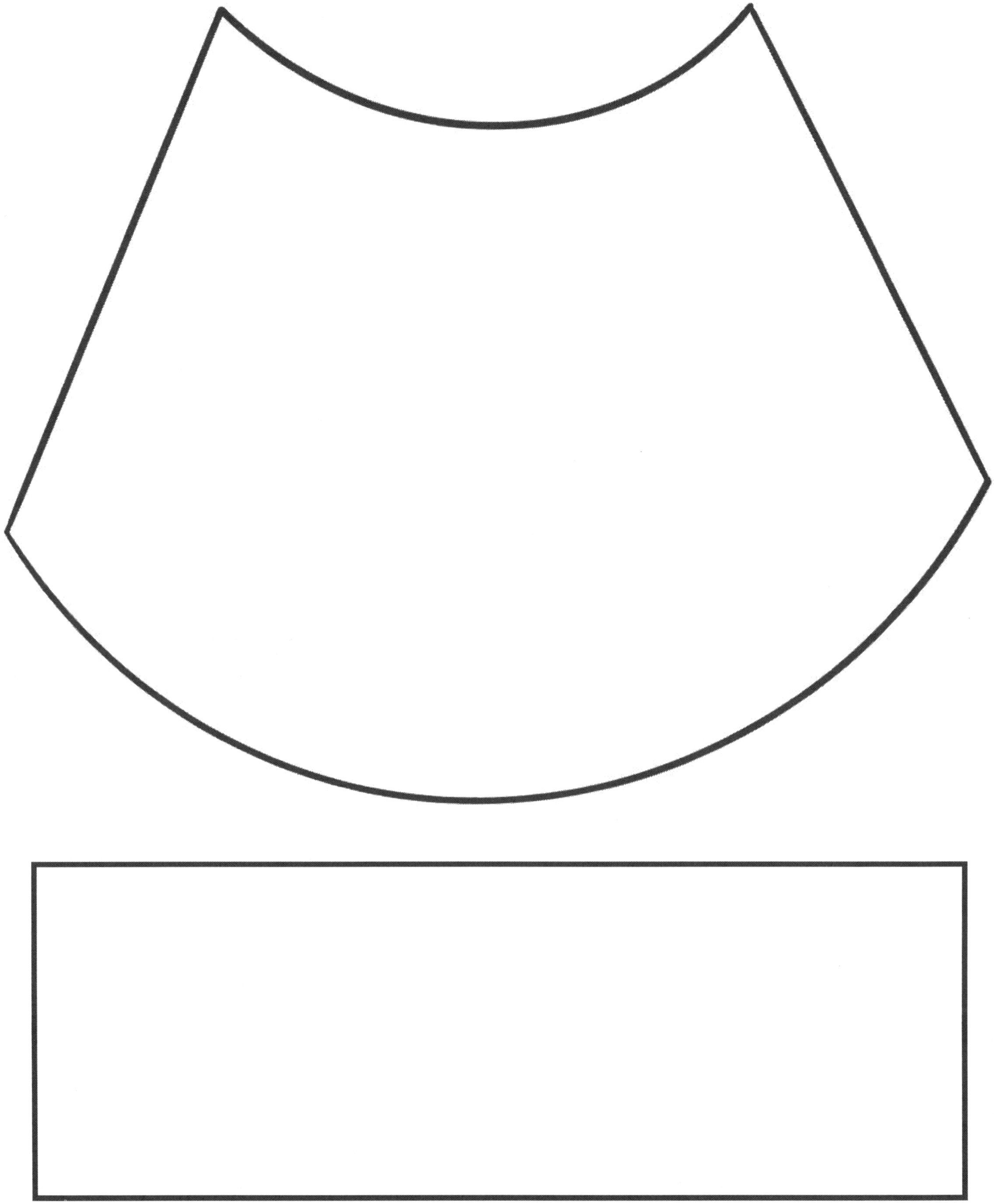

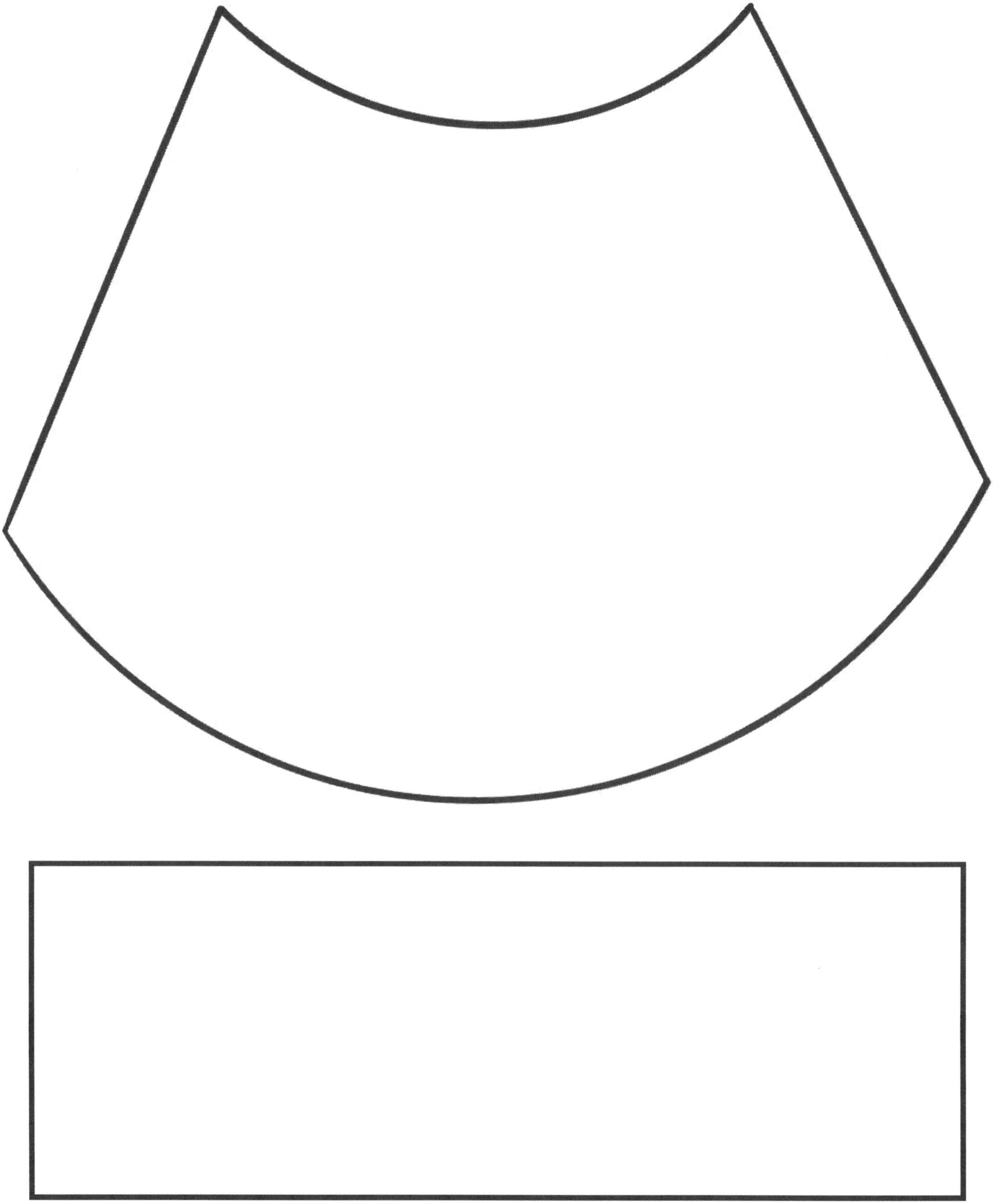

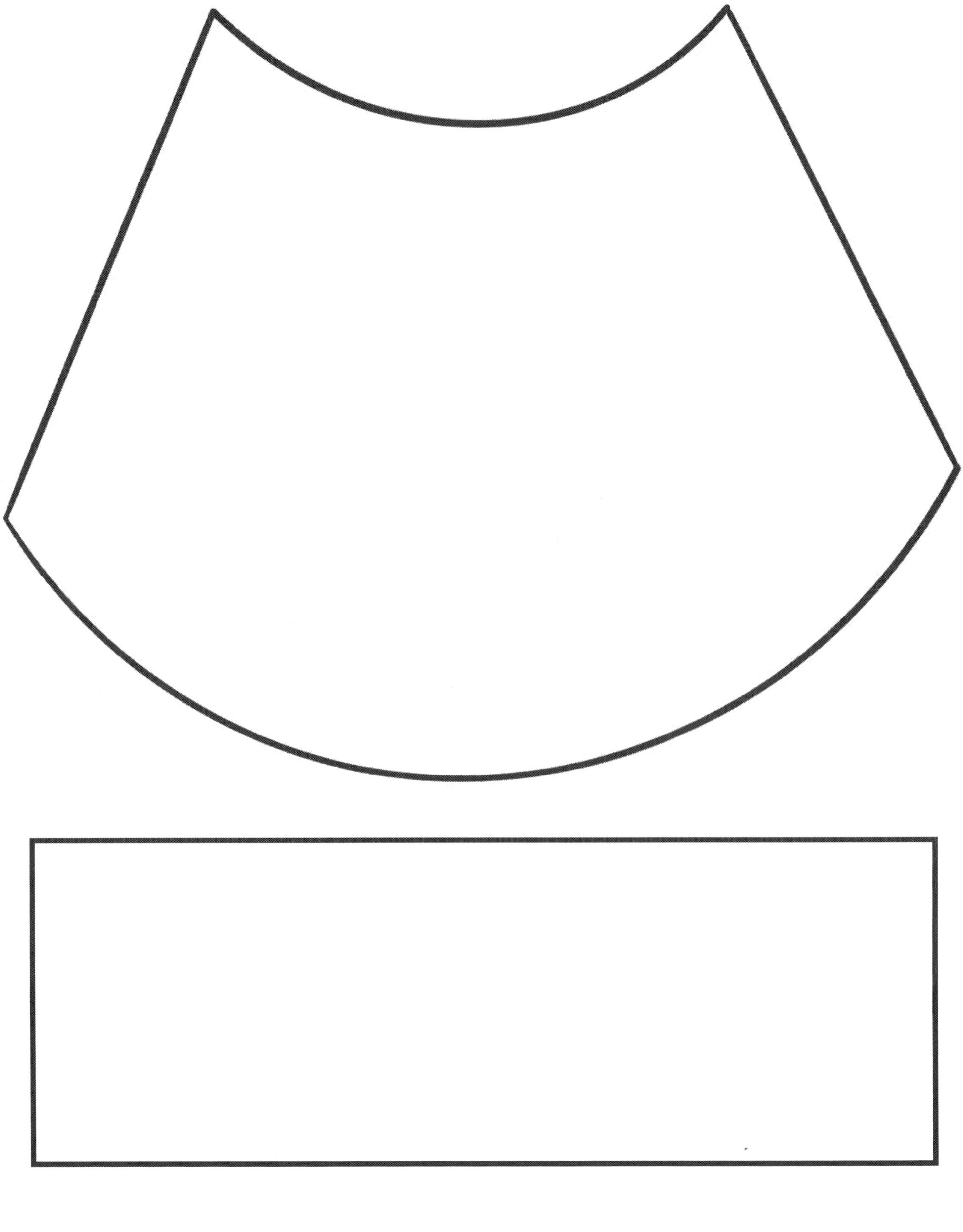

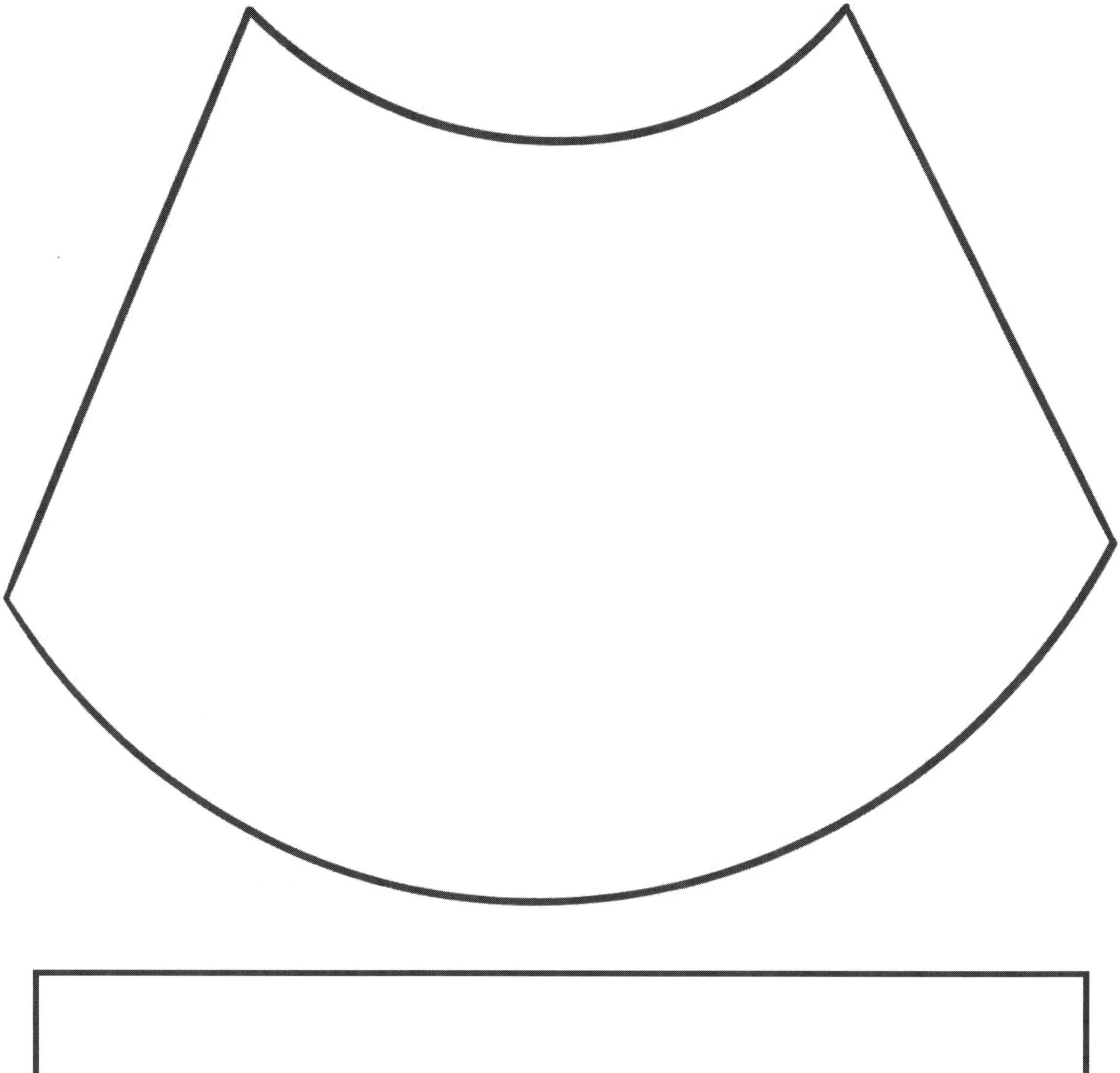

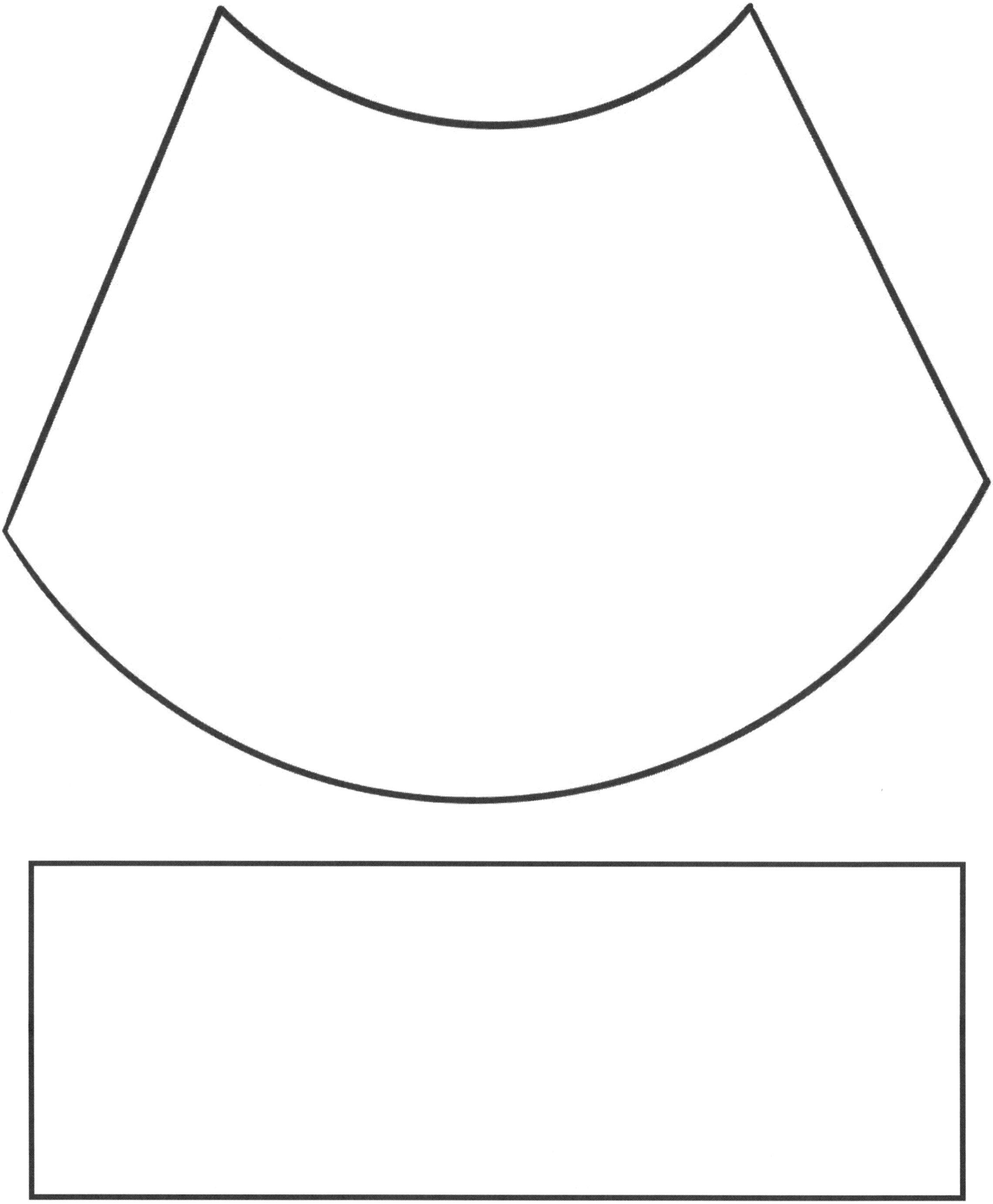

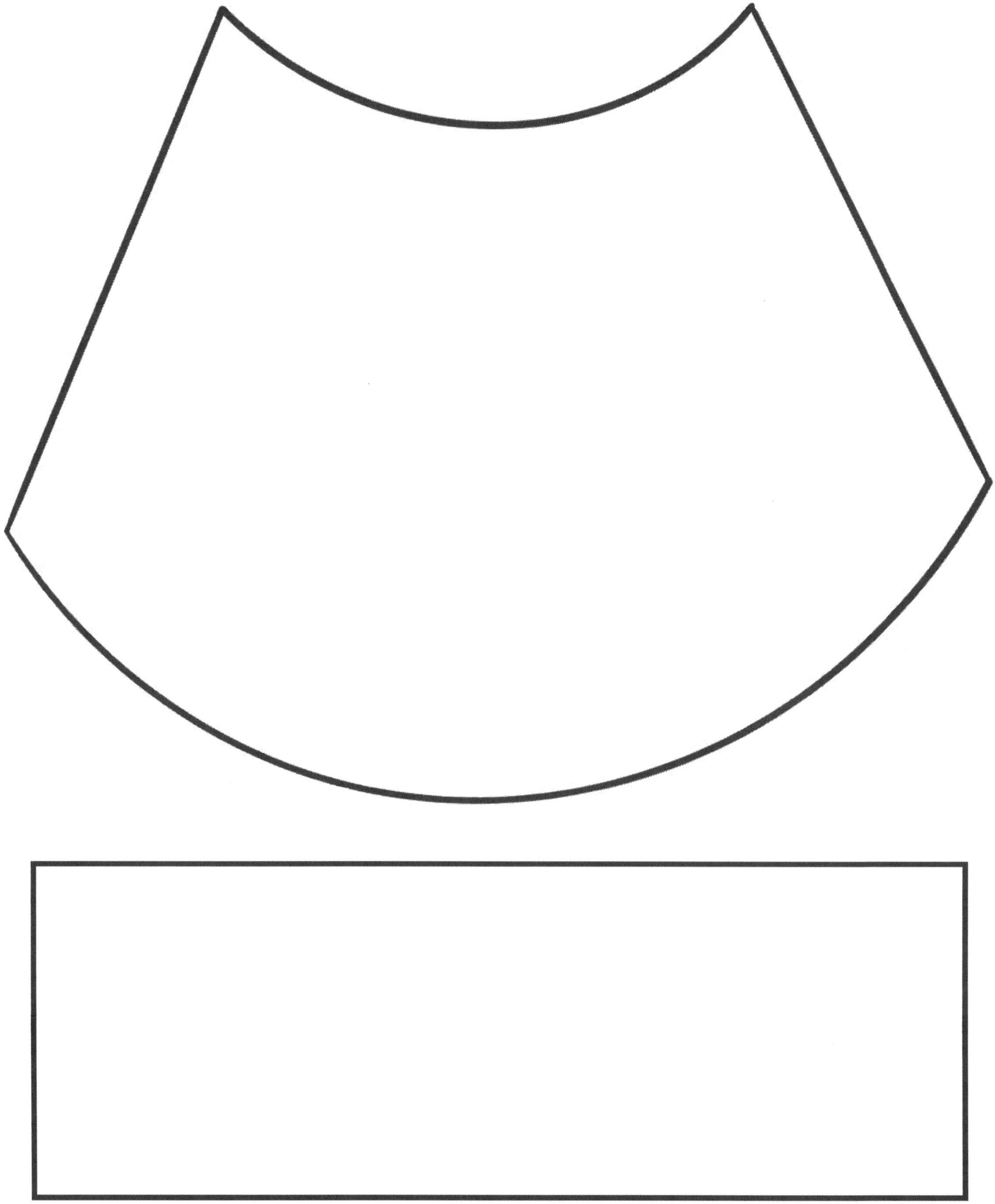

This page intentionally left blank

Made in the USA
Coppell, TX
28 December 2021

70323121R10068